So You Wanna Be a Yogi

So You Wanna Be a Yogi

A Guide to Becoming Yogarrific

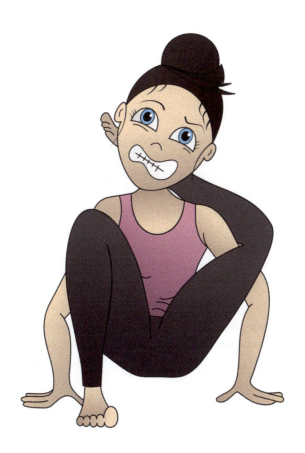

Presented by The Cartoon Yogi
Written and illustrated by

Krystel Dallas Houle

So You Wanna Be a Yogi

So You Wanna Be a Yogi is not intended as a substitute for the medical advice of physicians.

If you have medical concerns, please consult a physician before beginning a new exercise program. You should stop exercising immediately if you feel pain (the bad kind, not the "Geez, my abs are sure gonna feel this tomorrow!" kind), dizziness, or moderate to extreme discomfort. Always work within your own abilities and range of motion (Just because The Cartoon Yogi can bend any which way, doesn't mean you can or will ever be able to, and that's totally OK, because she's a cartoon, and I'm assuming that you're a real human person.)

The Cartoon Yogi shall not be held liable for any claims for injuries or damages resulting from the practice of the exercises or poses herein. (Also, careful, that coffee is hot.)

Cover design: Krystel Houle

Copyright © 2019 Krystel Houle
All rights reserved.

CONTENTS

ONE
Why You Should Do Yoga ~1

TWO
Why You Shouldn't Do Yoga ~4

THREE
It's More Than Just Pose ~12

FOUR
Class vs. Home Practice ~25

FIVE
Where to Start? ~41

SIX
Yoga Lingo ~53

SEVEN
Strike a Pose! ~56

EIGHT
Pranaya-wha? ~106

NINE
Bandhas ~114

TEN
Mantras, Mudras & Meditation ~119

ELEVEN
Chaka-Chaka-Chakras! ~141

TWELVE
Yoga Gear & Accessories ~145

THIRTEEN
Five Weird Things Yogis Say ~157

FOURTEEN
Eat Like a Yogi ~161

FIFTEEN
A Yogi's Quick Guide ~176

ONE

Why You Should Do Yoga

Why should you do yoga? Well…it

- helps you to relax;
- leaves you feeling more energetic;
- increases focus;
- reduces and manages stress;
- helps to balance your metabolism;
- strengthens and tones your muscles;
- improves your physical balance;
- increases your flexibility;
- improves your posture;
- hastens recovery from other sports;
- helps to prevent injury;
- can help with weight loss;
- improves circulation;
- can ease and help prevent arthritis;
- increases your joint range of motion;
- helps to strengthen bones and prevent osteoporosis;
- boosts immunity;
- can relieve depression;
- improves heart health;
- encourages a deeper sleep;
- can decrease pain in people with chronic conditions;
- improves your quality of life.

And the list goes on. Need I say more? OK, I will.

Yoga is the journey to true happiness. Even if you never make it there, there are so many benefits and great experiences to be had along the way that it's worth a try.

I've heard people say they hate yoga. Upon further investigation, most of these people had a bad experience in one class, with one teacher, and that turned them off of yoga entirely.

Well, friend, let me tell you there are many different types of yoga teachers out there, many different styles of yoga, and so much more to yoga than just poses. If you've had a bad experience, don't give up. With all of the benefits that yoga provides, it's worth another chance. Keep at it and you will find your tribe. Or maybe you won't. Maybe you'll be a lone wolf who practises on your own. That's cool too. Yoga is for everyone.

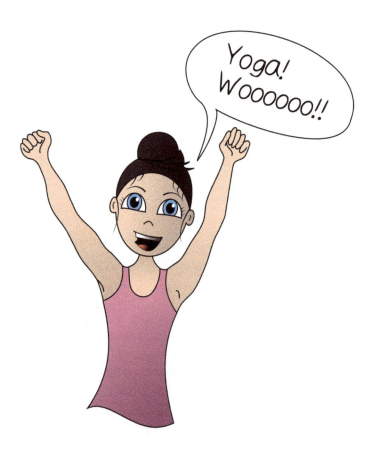

Whether you're a complete newbie, someone giving yoga another go, an occasional yogi who wants to practise more, or an experienced yogi who loves a refresher, we all have something to learn. We all have room for improvement.

We all have something to gain from yoga. There is a place for each of us in the yoga world.

So start today, even if it's just for five minutes. Don't put it off any longer.

Do it because it makes you happy.
Do it because it makes you feel good.
Do it because you love it.
Do it to become a better you.
Do it for me.

(Just kidding, you don't know me. Don't be weird.)

TWO

Why You Shouldn't Do Yoga

Myths & Misconceptions

Yoga is too easy.
Haha. HAHAhahaha! No. It's. Not. As you will see, yoga is a deep and complex practice. It could take a lifetime to master, if ever. Anything that can take a lifetime to master isn't easy. And if you're only interested in the physical benefits, trust me, you will be challenged there too. Anyone, at any level, can find ways to challenge themselves physically in yoga. If you've already tried a class and that's why you think it's too easy, then maybe you need to try a different class.

Yoga is too difficult.
It doesn't have to be. With all of the photos and videos we see on social media of advanced yogis showing us what they've got, it can be easy to think that. But there are so many beginner level poses that almost anyone can do. There's one where you just sit down with your legs criss-cross applesauce. It's called Easy Pose. Then, there's another one where you just lie there. Corpse Pose. In a beginner class, you won't be asked to do a headstand or anything too funky. If you are, you don't have to do it. Your yoga teacher is not a drill sergeant who is going to single you out and yell in your face if you're not doing what they say. Look for a style and level that suits where you're at right now and progress slowly, at your own pace.

Yoga is just for women.
Wrong. This currently female-dominated practice used to be a boys' club. It wasn't until the last hundred years that the number of yoginis began to grow. Some say that women were not allowed

to practise in the past. Some say that it was seen as improper for a woman to practise. Others say that women have always practised yoga. Whatever the case, what we do know is that today, when you go to a yoga class, there are typically way more girls than boys (if there are any boys at all). Over the past few decades, here in the West, yoga seems to have had the general reputation that it's a girly practice, that girls like to do, in their girly yoga pants and that it's too easy and girly for men to practise. Ha! In recent years, more and more men have been partaking in the fun and showing us what they've got. They are seeing for themselves that yoga is not for the faint. Men can benefit from the practice in the same way that women can, and in this day and age there is no reason that one gender should be dominating the practice more than the other.

Yoga is expensive.
It can be. If you like pretty things and have a shopping habit, then you are likely going to treat yourself to a bunch of new swag to go with your new passion. And classes can be expensive. But there are less expensive classes. The price of a class does not define its quality. Not to mention you can practise for free from home. All you need to start are comfy clothes and a mat. Maybe a hair elastic?

Yoga causes injuries.
Sure, if you're not careful. Don't attend an intermediate to advanced class if you're a beginner. Avoid a fast-paced flow if you have a back injury. You wouldn't go skiing for the first time down a black diamond hill...you'd start on the bunny hill. If a pose is painful, get out of it. Listen to your body and don't go beyond your own range of motion. This can be difficult for some people, especially in a class setting where they may find themselves competing with those around them. Remember, yoga is a practice, not a competition. You should always be in tune with how you feel in the moment and never push past your limits.

You can't get hurt doing yoga.
Yes, you can. That lady next to you who's twice your age and twisting herself into a pretzel? She's been practising for years and likes the pace of the beginner class you're attending. Just because she can do it, doesn't mean you can too. But you're gonna try, aren't ya? And you're gonna blow out your back and it's all because of yoga. You're going to miss work the next day and blame it on the class or on the teacher and then you're going to spend years telling people that you hate yoga because it injured your back. Yoga did. Not your ego. Yoga...

You have to chant in yoga class.
Do you? Some classes have chanting. Lots don't. If you don't want to chant, then don't. Be like the person at the birthday party who is just mouthing along to Happy Birthday while everyone else does all the singing. Except in yoga, you're not gonna get called out or poked fun at.

All yogis are vegan.
Not even at all. Some are. Some football players are vegan too. Sure, as yogis we practise love, compassion and non-violence towards ourselves and all living things and as a result many yogis choose to be vegetarian or vegan. However, this is not a requirement. There's no yoga club where the rules state that you can only be a member if you ditch the animal products. (There might be, I don't know.) Yoga is a personal practice, and the choices you make are yours.

All yogis are hippies.
Ahhhh hippies love yoga! But so do busy moms and stressed out corporate types. C'mon.

All yogis are bubbly, positive people.
OMG no. So many people go to yoga classes so that they can get away from the negativity and stress in life. You'll encounter all types, from the yogi suffering from mental illness who is there to improve their life, to the egocentric bitch who is there to show off.

Yogis are regular people like you and me. Yes, you'll also run into the odd person who is seemingly always positive and bubbly, but those people have something to hide...Muah ha ha!

Yoga teachers can do all the poses.
Nope. Each yogi has poses that they excel at, and those they can't do, and may never be able to do. Our bodies are all shaped differently. That means that something that is easy for one person may not be easy for the next, yoga teacher or not. We also may have had injuries that prevent us from moving certain ways. Yoga teachers are not immune to this and they certainly understand that their students have limitations as well.

Yogis are all spiritual.
Nuh-uh. As individuals, we get to choose how deeply we want to delve into the world of yoga. Most people will be partaking in the poses and some meditation and that's it. How in tune you are with your spiritual side is a very personal thing. You won't be judged if you don't like the spirituality of yoga and don't want to incorporate it into your practice. With time, some bits and pieces of it may filter into your life naturally. And if not, fine. And if the super spiritual types in class bother you, move your mat over so that they're not beside you. If it's the teacher, try a different class. There are plenty of classes out there that focus on yoga as exercise or that take a more straightforward approach.

Yogis can't drink alcohol.
Ever been to class hungover? I have. It is not fun. As yogis, we are encouraged to practise self-control. As humans, we sometimes lose control. On purpose. This is not a rule. It's just something you may want to avoid the night before an early morning class...

Yoga is just glorified stretching.
Well, it's not JUST glorified stretching. It's also glorified strength training. And glorified stamina building. And a glorified balancing act. A physical, mental, emotional and spiritual practice with glorified benefits. Yoga is glorious.

Yoga is a religion.
It's not a religion. It's not a cult. It's a lifestyle. Practised by people of various religious backgrounds and by people with no religious beliefs.

Excuses, Excuses

I'm too old.
This can actually be an advantage. When beginning a yoga practice, it's important to be patient and listen to our bodies. These are things we tend to get better at with age. As we age, we tend to do more things for ourselves, to improve our quality of life. In this way, we are less likely to become competitive with those around us and more likely to focus on our own practice. As a result, we reap the benefits much quicker. No matter what age you are, choosing the right class is essential for a safe and enjoyable experience. Beginner classes, Restorative Yoga, Yoga for the Elderly (assuming you actually are old and not some middle-aged person who just thinks they're old but isn't) there's something for everyone in yoga. Still not ready to try the poses? Practise meditation. Don't forget, that's yoga too.

I'm too big.
No, you're not. Yoga is not about having a perfect body. Yoga is for *every*body. Being a low-impact physical practice, it's perfect for anyone worried about their joints when they exercise. Not only that, but it also helps to strengthen the stabilizing muscles surrounding your joints, making everyday tasks easier on your body. There are ways to modify and vary poses to accommodate everyone in a yoga class. And if you're not comfortable with a certain pose, just don't do it. You won't be judged for going to class with the goal of improving your life. That's what the other yogis are there for too. And if you do get judged, then it's those jerks who don't belong there, not you. If you're uncomfortable being in a class, try starting your practice at home. With time,

you'll develop balance, strength, flexibility and confidence that will serve you in everything you do.

I'm not flexible enough.
Flexibility isn't the only thing practised in yoga. Strength, balance and stamina are all a part of it too. Some people excel more at one thing than another. By practising, your flexibility will improve over time. Flexibility is certainly not required to start a yoga practice. Remember, not everyone looks the same holding the same pose. We're all made and shaped differently and that is reflected in our physical practices. You wouldn't wait to be able to do handstand push-ups to start going to CrossFit classes. Don't wait to be flexible to start a yoga practice.

I have a bad back.
Let your instructor know. This way they can offer you variations of poses so that you can have a safe and enjoyable experience. Find a class in a studio, or online, that is geared to back pain. Move slowly and carefully. Listen to your body and avoid poses that make you feel worse. A regular practice can improve your mobility and quality of life.

I have arthritis.
Yoga has been proven to help those with arthritis reduce joint pain and increase their range of motion. The key is to find the style and class that is right for you. If you are practising from home, look for sequences geared towards your condition. If you're in a class and it is not specifically for those suffering from arthritis, let the instructor know before you begin so that they may offer any variations they think can improve your experience.

The women there will think I'm a perv.
If you're a dude who strategically positions himself in a class where he can ogle all the pretty ladies, and then proceeds to do just that making those around him uncomfortable, then yeah, the women are gonna think you're a perv. But a man who shows up to a yoga class, with the intention of getting in a solid practice, acts

respectful and genuine, then no. No one is going to think you're attending yoga because you're a perv. Yoga is for everyone, not just women. Most women are happy to see men attend class. It can even encourage them to up their game and prove to themselves that they're just as a strong as their male counterparts. Because women are. If a woman doesn't want to practise in the same room as a man, she will attend an all-female class. Just be cool, OK?

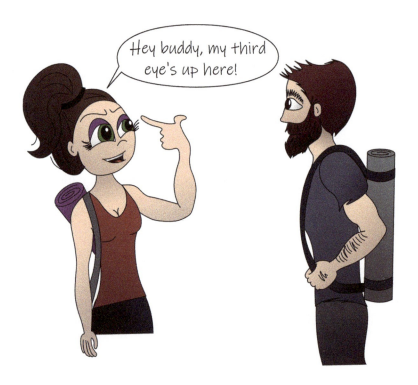

I sweat too much.
Bah! Bring a towel. No one will mind unless you're sending sweat spray over to your neighbour. If anything, people will think you worked harder than they did!

I don't know the poses.
It's called a yoga *class*. Where you *practise* yoga. Classes are where you go to learn things. Go often enough and you'll pick it up. If you don't, just pretend and do what the person beside you is doing.

I don't have time.
Really? You don't have 15 minutes to follow a video at home? How much time are you spending on your phone or on social media every day? Can some of that time be afforded to a little thing called self-care? You don't need to leave your house to practise yoga. And you don't have to practise for hours at a time to experience the benefits. Some poses in the morning. A bit of meditation before bed. You're doing it. You're a yogi.

I don't like yoga.
Bullshit! You don't like breathing properly? You don't like having control over your body, mind and emotions? You don't like a quiet moment to yourself? In yoga, there is something for everyone. If you had a bad experience, move on. Switch it up. You'll find something that suits you. Just because you didn't like a certain pasta dish doesn't mean you don't like pasta. There are different types of pasta. And different sauces. And toppings. And settings in which to consume them. Think about it. Makes sense, right?

THREE

It's More Than Just Poses

When you think of yoga, you may think of postures (poses), or a class full of limber bodies in various positions with their mats rolled out getting their stretch on. You may even think of someone seated in meditation.

Poses or asanas are just one limb out of eight, or one branch out of six, that make up what yoga is. In the West, much of the focus is on the physical side of yoga. That isn't to say that that's all we do. Many instructors include the other aspects of yoga in their teachings, and many yogis work them into their daily practice. However, with our busy schedules and stress-filled lives, we often seek to "Zen out" as quickly as possible, fitting a yoga class in on our lunch hour or between appointments. And because many students are seeking the physical feeling and benefits that yoga postures provide, classes will often focus only on that. There's nothing wrong with that, it's just that there is so much more to yoga than just poses.

The way we see and think of yoga is greatly influenced by the media. Ads feature svelte bodies donning expensive "yoga" apparel, sometimes posed in a position that isn't really a yoga asana at all. Posters for classes may show a full class or just one person striking an impressive, advanced posture. And not to mention all of the attention yogis get on social media, like Instagram, by posting beautiful photos of themselves and their practice, some before and after photos, and tips. It's no wonder a non-yogi wouldn't really know that yoga is so much more than all of that. As you'll see, it would be pretty difficult to capture it all in a photograph.

So what is yoga?

If you look up the definition of yoga, you will be presented with so many different answers you won't know which holds true. It is defined differently by region, by religion, and by source. In Sanskrit, the word yoga means "union" and by its origin means "to join, to unite, to control, to discipline".

Yoga is a way of life. Yoga is a spiritual, mental and physical self-discipline which includes practising meditation, moderation, breath control and physical postures, increasing self-awareness, and control of body and mind. Its purpose is to find your own path to enlightenment.

Yoga is a very personal practice, individual to each yogi. In exploring these different areas, forms, branches or limbs of yoga we can really see why. As a beginner, you may want to start with simple classes, learning the postures. I do think it is important, however, to know a bit more if you want to call yourself a yogi. I will give a brief description of a few of the vast areas you can explore. From there, you can personalize your practice to suit yourself.

The Six Branches of Yoga

There are six commonly recognized branches of yoga: raja, hatha, jnana, bhakti, karma and tantra. Each of these branches is complex and many go on to explore further sub-branches or "twigs". Just kidding, no one calls them that.

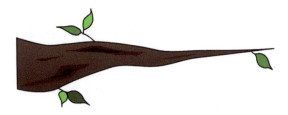

Raja Yoga: yoga of the mind, or the Royal Path. Raja yoga focuses on the mind and meditation. This branch is linked to and follows the eight limbs of Patanjali.

Hatha Yoga: the physical practice of yoga. Any yoga class that we attend or form of yoga we do where postures are practised is Hatha yoga, whether it be a Vinyasa yoga class, Power yoga, Hot yoga, etc. The purpose of Hatha yoga is to calm the body by freeing it of limitations, therefore calming the mind and spirit to prepare for meditation.

Jnana Yoga: the yoga of wisdom and knowledge. Considered a difficult practice, Jnana yoga focuses on the study of yoga scriptures and philosophical texts. It is the practice of self-reflection, self-realization, with goals of liberating oneself of ego and attachment to material possessions. Ultimately, to liberate oneself of suffering.

Bhakti Yoga: the yoga of devotion (and chanting). Bhakti yoga is selfless. It is the surrender to the divine, or a higher being. It is love and respect, tolerance and acceptance for all beings, regardless of what you believe.

Karma Yoga: the yoga of action. Karma yoga is the act of doing things for the betterment of others, without desire for personal gain. It is selfless service that is free from negativity. Practised with the notion that our existence today is influenced by the decisions we made in the past, or simply: what goes around comes around. In other words, karma is only a bitch if you are.

Tantra Yoga: the yoga of weaving (or expansion, awakening). Though your mind may make a sexual connection when hearing the term, it is much more than an intense sexual experience. That type of experience, however, can be achieved as a result of practising Tantra yoga. In combining the other branches of yoga, we develop such a strong connection to self that we increase our well-being, mindfulness, confidence and strength. Tantra yoga gives us a sense of bliss.

The Four Paths of Yoga

You may not have heard of The Four Paths of Yoga. Different religions, regions and groups follow different combinations of yogic philosophies. One such combination is The Four Paths of Yoga. Similar to The Six Branches of Yoga, The Four Paths include: Karma Yoga, Bhakti Yoga, Raja Yoga and Gyana (Jnana) Yoga.

While they differ in that they do not include Hatha or Tantra Yoga, The Four Paths of Yoga and The Six Branches of Yoga have ultimately the same goal. By combining focuses, one can achieve bliss, happiness, contentment, self-awareness and enlightenment.

The Eight Limbs of Yoga (as described by Patanjali)

"Yoga takes you into the present moment, the only place where life exists." - Patanjali

Yoga dates back 5000+ years, originating from the Vedas which are ancient Hindu scriptures and texts. Asanas weren't even part of the original show. Now we know the yoga we practise today began in the 2nd century BC. A sage named Patanjali summarized his yogic knowledge to create the Yoga Sutras and to define what we know today as The Eight Limbs of Yoga. And even so, it wasn't until about 800 years later that yoga postures made their appearance into our regular practice.

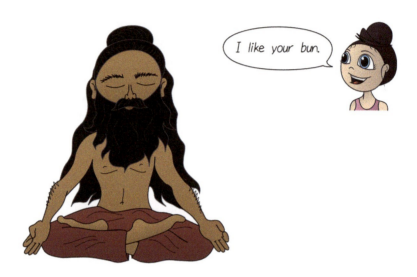

Patanjali created The Eight Limbs to help us go beyond the confines of our ego to achieve self-realization. As humans, boy do we suffer. We have emotions, desires, expectations, needs, goals, failures, relationships, jobs (am I right?), which all cause us to suffer. Yoga was created as a way for us to rise above our suffering. It teaches us to let go of our attachment to material belongings. It teaches us to live a more disciplined life with the goal to achieve enlightenment. Through yoga practice we can become one with the divine, a higher being, something bigger than us. Through practice we learn to live fully, to be real. We grow to know who we are and what our purpose is. We stop the endless search for life's answers as we begin to find those answers within us.

Ashtanga yoga (ashta = eight, ang = limb) is a popular yoga term you may have heard. Ashtanga yoga is the style of yoga whose practitioners focus on the Eight Limbs as described by Patanjali.

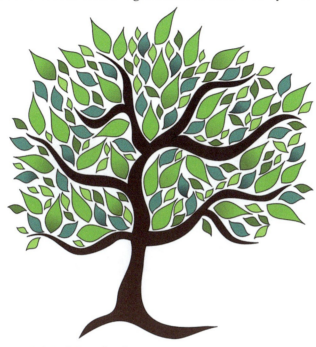

1. <u>Yamas</u>: Ethical Standards

There are five Yamas:
- Ahimsa: to be non-violent, to be compassionate
- Satya: to be truthful
- Asteya: to not steal
- Bramacharya: to be self-aware, to have self-control
- Aparigraha: to not be greedy, to be non-possessive

The Yamas pertain to how we relate to those around us. Our integrity and moral code are examined and refined. The Yamas remind us to be a good person all the time, wherever we go. Not just when we're sitting on our yoga mat.

To practise: Begin with the first Yama and put a special focus on it for a week. Keep a journal of moments that stand out during that week, good or bad, and describe what you can do to improve this Yama. After a week, add the 2nd Yama, and so on.

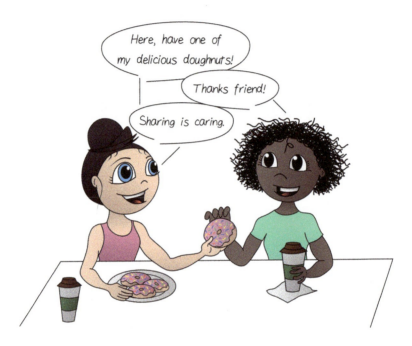

2. Niyamas: Personal Standards/Self-Discipline

There are five Niyamas:
- Saucha: to be pure of body, speech and mind
- Santosha: to be content, satisfied
- Tapas: to be modest, disciplined, committed
- Svadhyaya: to study sacred/philosophical texts, to practise self-study, to be introspective
- Ishvara Pranidhana: to be devoted to a higher power, to surrender to your spirituality

The Niyamas relate to our relationship with ourselves. They encourage us to improve our self-behaviour, our self-discipline, our self-awareness and our self-study. The Niyamas remind us that it's important to think and reflect on what we say and do, and also what we don't say and don't do.

To practise: Begin with the first Niyama and put a special focus on it for a week. Keep a journal of moments that stand out during that week, good or bad, and describe what you can do to improve this Niyama. After a week, add the 2nd Niyama, and so on.

3. **Asana**: Posture

Asanas are the physical poses that form part of our yoga practice.

The word asana in Sanskrit translates to "seat". It's believed that in its origin, the only pose practised in yoga was the seat you take in meditation. With time, more poses were developed to aid in the aches one gets after sitting for long periods of time. This ended up being beneficial in preparing the body and mind for the meditative state by allowing the practitioner to master their physical body in order to sit still for meditation. Now, we have a multitude of poses that provide a wide range of benefits.

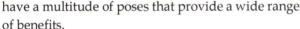

In practising asanas, we can increase our flexibility, build physical strength, improve our physical and mental balance, detoxify our organs, reduce stress, eliminate toxins and improve our blood circulation.

Practising yoga asanas prepares the body for the remaining Yoga Sutras: Pranayama, Pratyahara, Dharana, Dhyana and Samadhi.

To practise: Begin a physical practice three days/week even for just 15 minutes at a time. Over time, increase the duration and/or frequency of your practice until you are practising every day.

4. Pranayama: Breathing Techniques

Pranayama is the expansion of our vital life force through breathing exercises. It is our breath.

When we experience negative emotions such as stress, anger, anxiety or fear, our breath may become erratic, beyond our control, even restricted (think: panic attack). Pranayama helps us to overcome this. By controlling our breath, we learn to control our mind, guiding it to a state of stillness or peace thereby restoring our breath to a state of ease.

Practising breathing techniques in yoga allows us to expand our energy and go beyond what we believe ourselves to be physically and mentally capable of. When practising an asana for example, say Warrior II, we may feel the need to get out of the pose when it becomes difficult. Once our legs start to burn and shake, we begin to restrict or hold our breath and our mind tells us to let go. Being aware of this and turning our focus to controlling and slowing down our breath in this type of situation allows us to hold the pose for a longer time. This same practice can be applied to everyday life when things become difficult, to help us gain control in a situation.

To practise: Start by simply being aware of your breath. Notice if and when it changes, becomes restricted. And notice when it feels the most natural and at ease. Recognize the situations or thoughts that create these changes.

5. Pratyahara: Sensory Withdrawal

An important preparatory stage for meditation, pratyahara is the practice of withdrawing from external stimulation. The five senses provide distractions, particularly sound, although everybody is different. Through this practice, we become unaffected by external stimuli, shifting our focus to our inner selves.

To practise: Turn off the TV, put your phone on silent, shut off your computer and any other sounds that you can. Close your eyes and sit in silence for one full minute. If that was easy, try five minutes. If you have kids, have them do it too! They may only last 10 seconds to start, and that's OK!

Note: Sensory deprivation tanks are becoming popular, especially for athletes, allowing them to heal their mind and body from the strains and stresses of their sport. A quick search online will let you know if any spas in your area provide this service.

6. Dharana: Concentration

Taking us one step closer to meditation, dharana is the practice of eliminating internal distractions, bringing our focus to a single point for a calm and still mind. That point of focus may be a mantra (a sound, word or phrase that is repeated over and over for the duration of the exercise or meditation session), a symbol or an object.

Having already worked on eliminating external distractions through our practice of pratyahara, we must now rid our minds of thoughts, emotions, colours, shapes or images that may interfere with our concentration. Should your attention sway to a distraction, simply become aware of it, and return to your mantra. The more we concentrate on our mantra, the stronger our focus becomes, the quicker we can get back there.

To practise: Choose a sound (example: om), word, mantra, affirmation, symbol or object that will be your point of internal focus. Aim for something positive. Sit in Easy Pose (cross-legged) or a seated posture that is comfortable to you, with your eyes closed, hands on your knees or folded in your lap. Repeat your word, mantra or affirmation over and over either out loud, in a humming fashion, or silently to yourself for several minutes. For symbols and objects, envision them. If your focus begins to wander, simply return your concentration to your original point of focus.

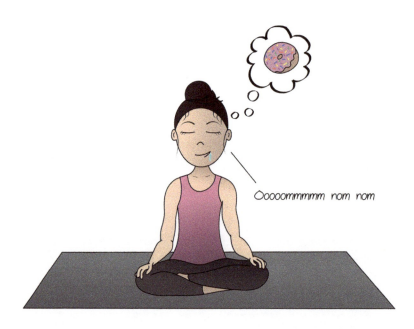

7. Dhyana: Meditation

Now that we've been practising the six previous limbs, we are ready to meditate! As you may have deduced, dharana naturally leads to meditation. In dharana, we are strongly and intentionally concentrating on our point of focus. In meditation, we become one with our mantra. Our focus becomes effortless. We have moments of pure stillness, where the body and mind are focusing on nothing at all. We notice no distractions. We have few to no thoughts and when we do, we eliminate them, effortlessly returning to our mantra and then to stillness. Because of this, we may waver between dharana and dhyana throughout our practice.

The purpose of meditation is to relax and find peace. Meditation leads us to samadhi, which is the place you really want to go, but never knew you did, so you'll be ecstatic when you get there...if you ever do.

To practise: Sit in Easy Pose (cross-legged) or a seated posture that is comfortable to you, with your hands on your knees or folded in your lap away from external distractions as much as possible. You can close your eyes or light a candle and place it in front of you where you will maintain your gaze (dhristi). Begin with a slow and steady breath (pranayama), followed by shutting out external senses (pratyahara), then begin to repeat your mantra to yourself silently, bringing all of your focus to your mantra (dharana). If your mind wanders, return your focus to your mantra for several minutes. As you become more relaxed, stop repeating your mantra and allow your body and mind to sit in stillness and silence. Start with just five minutes/day.

8. Samadhi: Pure Consciousness

This is the big one! The one that all of our practice leads us to. Samadhi. Ultimate Bliss. Enlightenment. Ecstasy. Nirvana. Where in dhyana we become one with our mantra, in samadhi we become one with the divine, with a higher power, a supreme state of consciousness. Samadhi is a trance-like state in which we are in a complete state of effortless concentration. An oxymoron, I know. This is the goal of yoga. Should this state be elusive though, fret not. Many yogis will never experience true samadhi.

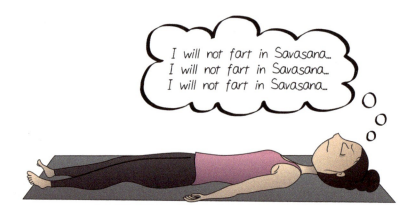

To practise: Following meditation, lay back in Savasana (see chapter 7), surrender your thoughts, allow yourself to sink into a deeper meditative state. If you get jerked back to reality, it's because you were falling asleep. That's OK, happens to the best of us.

FOUR

Class vs. Home Practice

So you've made up your mind, you're giving yoga a go. Or maybe you've been dabbling in it and want a more consistent practice. It's time to find the setting that's right for you. Class or home practice?

In Class Practice

Class settings can vary from studio classes, private classes for you and a few friends, to classes offered at community centres, the YMCA, martial arts clubs, health clubs, dance studios, etc.

If you're looking at jumping into a public class, it can be intimidating seeing all that is offered. Especially if the studio or club you're looking at has come up with clever and original names for their classes. Typically if this studio or club has a website, a description of each class will be included. If you're a beginner to yoga, look for a class that is suitable to you, or try a general class.

In a general class, the teacher must expect that there will be beginners participating and will be able to spot you. Simply because they haven't seen you there before, they will keep an eye on you to gauge what level you're at. If you're still not sure where to start, talk to the receptionist or a teacher at the studio. You will find they can be quite helpful and encouraging.

Whether you are new to yoga or not, it's always a good idea to introduce yourself to the instructor before or after a class that is new-to-you. Normally you need to sign a waiver and fill out a form outlining any previous experience and injuries before attending a public class, however, in many cases, the instructor will not have a chance to read through your form before the class starts. If you have a specific injury or other issue that can benefit from specific modifications, let the teacher know. If you don't let the teacher know, you may have a bad experience that could have been avoided. Knowing about your issue in advance, a good instructor will pay close attention to you during parts of the class that can negatively affect your condition, and provide modifications, variations and support to ensure you have a positive experience.

Don't be shy to ask questions. Yoga instructors love helping people and guiding them through their journey. If you don't communicate concerns, or ask questions about the things that are confusing or bothering you, that bad experience you may have can been avoided. While your instructors will do what they can to provide a pleasant experience for everyone, they don't always have the time to stop and converse with each participant in their class. Especially when the number of participants is high or their class schedules are packed. Speak up.

That being said, there are certain times and ways to explore or speak up to ensure that you, and those around you, enjoy the class. It's a sort of unspoken etiquette that as yogis, we must follow so that we don't come off as inconsiderate assholes.

Yoga Class Etiquette

Show up on time: Aim to arrive to class 5 to 10 minutes before it is scheduled. Even earlier if you need to pay for the class beforehand or have a word with the instructor. Expect that a class will start on time. And if you do need to walk into a class after it's started, do so quietly and position yourself near the back.

Don't snap your mat: Some people unroll their mats by grabbing either corner of the short edge and whipping their mat out to lay it flat, like when people with long arms put sheets on their beds. If whipped out hard enough, the mat will make a snapping sound. This is annoying for everyone and startling to most. Particularly those who are stretching or practising breathing techniques before class starts. Don't. Snap. Your. Mat.

Don't disrupt if you have to leave early: If you must leave early for whatever reason, try to do so as quietly as possible, without stepping over other people on your way out. Ideally, set up your mat near the door.

Don't compete with others: Yoga is a practice, not a competition. The same pose will look different on different bodies. Just because someone looks to be doing a pose differently than you are, it's not necessarily better or worse. They may be at a different level than you. Their bones may be shaped differently than yours. They might actually be doing it wrong and are about to get injured. Pay others no mind. Listen to the teacher's instructions and focus on yourself.

Be aware of your stuff: If you must bring things into class with you (water bottle, cell phone, towel, sweater, etc.), keep them close to your mat, away from your neighbours and out of the path between mats, that people use to walk past you.

Cell phones: If you bring your cell phone to class, turn it off. The sound of a phone on vibrate is just as distracting as a low ringtone. Even if your phone is stuffed away in your purse. If you have to have your phone out because you may be expecting an emergency call (a house deal, your wife's going into labour, etc.), then let the instructor know beforehand that your phone will be out in front of you because you may have to take it. In this case, position yourself near the door so that you can sneak out if you have to take a call.

Stay off the mat: Other people's mats, that is. Throughout your practice you will be all over your mat. Even your face will touch down on it. You wouldn't want to have other people's footprints right under your nose, so keep yours off of other people's mats.

Shoes/Tidiness: No shoes. No socks either. If studio floors irk you and you don't want to be barefoot anywhere but on your mat, come prepared with some indoor slip-ons or some yoga-specific socks. Also, knowing you're going to be barefoot, try to make sure your feet aren't dirty or stinky...

Practice cleanliness: Haven't had a chance to shower in a while? Been sweating a lot today? Forgot your deodorant? Smelling a little rank? Might be a good idea to skip class and practise at home. The heat from the class and the sweat you'll build up will make you smell worse to yourself and others, which can be very distracting.

Sweat spray: Are you a super-sweater? When practising dynamic movements and quick transitions, be conscious if you're sending sweat droplets over to your neighbours. If you know this might happen, bring a towel and dab yourself off every now and then throughout the practice.

Strong odours: That perfume you put on this morning? It may smell stronger to others than to you. Skip the perfume when going to class if you can. Hair products and strong-smelling lotions as well. Smoker? Maybe don't light up right before class. Sweating brings out odours and makes them stronger. Had some drinks last night? That alcohol smell will come right through your pores. So try not to binge the night before a morning class. Got it?

Chewing gum: Just don't.

Sniffles/Coughing: While you might avoid class regularly when you're sick, it sometimes creeps up on you and you can't help it. Most classes, studios or clubs will have tissues available. Keep a few at the top corner of your mat if you need to blow your nose. Keep a water bottle nearby in case you have to cough. Position yourself near the back of the class in case you need to walk out to get through a coughing fit. Try to be as non-distracting as possible.

Wear appropriate attire: I see London, I see France, I see Yogi's underpants! Your pants might not seem see-through when you're checking yourself out in the mirror, but bend over and that material stretching over your butt might just expose your goods. Keep that in mind if you're gonna wear a thong. You may not care, but other people might, especially if you're attending a general class where children are welcome. Also, pay attention to what you're wearing on top. Ladies, is your bra supportive? Or is downward dog gonna cause a nip slip...something to consider. Some clubs/studios might require full tops in their classes, find out if there's a dress code before signing up, or come prepared.

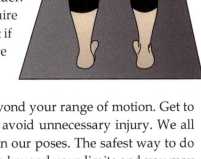

Know your limits: Don't go beyond your range of motion. Get to know your limits and you will avoid unnecessary injury. We all want to progress and advance in our poses. The safest way to do so is slowly and with control. Go beyond your limits and you may slip on your mat, fall over or pop something out of place.

Respect other people's space: If space is tight and you're in close proximity to the person next to you, you may end up getting in each other's way during certain poses. Pay attention to where they are and try to stagger yourselves so that you don't hit each other.

Don't be a loud mouth: Ujjayi breath aside, grunting and making struggling sounds during a class means you're working too hard. That's not what yoga is about. If you have to struggle through a class, you may have chosen a class that is too advanced for you. Deep breathing is fine, and is expected, however exaggerated breathing should be kept for times when the class is doing pranayama together.

Giggling buddies: Going to class with a friend? Maybe one that doesn't exercise, thinks yoga is stupid and is just going for fun...sure, it can be funny when your friend is having a tough go and making struggling faces on purpose to make you laugh. Or maybe you're whispering to each other and being silly. This is super distracting not only to the other yogis attending class, but especially to the teacher. Take the class seriously. It's not to say you can't go together and have a good time, you did pay for the class after all. So did everyone else though. And they're not getting their money's worth if you and your buddy are making asses of yourselves. If you can't follow a class side by side without disrupting, then you might want to find another activity to do together.

Don't go rogue: The class is in Extended Side Angle and you want to progress to a Bind & Twist? That's totally fine. But the class is in Extended Side Angle and you want to do Dancer Pose? Don't. Respect the instructor's class sequence. It's fine to do a variation of a pose that the class is already doing. You will see that a lot. You may even see someone holding Mountain Pose or Child's Pose if they're not comfortable with the pose being done and want to avoid it. That's fine too. Those are still poses, that will not distract anyone. But taking your own liberties can be. If you don't like to follow a class, practise at home.

Don't linger too long: Chances are there's another class coming in after yours or your instructor has somewhere to be. Most will give themselves time after class to talk and see their yogis out. This is a great time to ask any questions or give updates to your instructor. Maybe after class you want to chat with other yogis. That's great! But don't be the guest that just won't leave. Pick up your stuff, say what you have to say and get out of the class. You can always continue your conversation outside.

While most of these practices seem like common sense, not everyone will follow them. Be ready for anything. There are all types of yogis that you're likely to encounter.

Types of Yogis

The rogue yogi: someone who does what poses they want regardless of what the class is doing.

The yoga bitch: that person who has all the fancy expensive yoga gear and only does yoga because they think it makes them look cool.

The show-off who's not trying to show off: they take advanced variations of a lot of the poses in the class because it feels good and they're just at that level.

The show-off who is trying to show off: they take advanced variations of a lot of the poses in the class because they want you to know how good they are.

The know-it-all: easy to spot, they'll pipe up when they think they know different than the teacher or feel it necessary to add something.

The confused yogi: the instructor says turn right, they turn left. More complicated instructions might leave them with a blank stare while they awkwardly try to figure out how to move.

The yogi-in-a-hurry: quick to transition and restless holding a pose, the first one up from savasana and the first to roll up their mat and scurry off when class is barely done.

The loud breather: you can hear them from a mile away.

The free spirit: they place their mat askew, they smell of patchouli and give off the best vibes, man.

The friendly yogi: they talk to everyone and are super approachable, making you feel super welcome.

The sleepy yogi: they're the one who's snoring in savasana.

The gassy yogi: whoever smelled it dealt it.

The loner yogi: they keep to themselves, they sneak in and out, you don't even know they're there.

Sometimes a yogi will fall under two or more of these categories during the same class. It's important to be aware of how you feel about these people and how you feel when someone goes against class etiquette. This will help you make a conscious effort every time you attend a class, to ensure the experience is enjoyable not only for yourself, but also for those around you (by not being a jerk).

Some people will not fall under any of these categories. We're human, we're an odd bunch always finding new ways to be weird and annoy each other.

I'd like to take a moment to acknowledge the gassy yogi. There may be a day when that yogi is you and there will certainly be a day when that yogi is beside you. Ignore it. Everyone else probably will too. Or laugh it off. It's pretty funny. Just be cool about it. Don't judge. Farting is good for you.

While the thought of sharing space with a group of potential weirdos may not appeal to you at first, there is something to be said about the motivation that a group setting provides. For example, let's say that you only practise yoga at home. If on this particular day, you'd really rather just be lazy than stick to your practice, you may skip your workout entirely, falsely convincing yourself that you'll make up for it later. By showing up to class whether you feel like it or not, you will go through the motions and feel better for it when you're done. After all, you'd look pretty silly just sitting there, not moving, while everyone else goes through the poses!

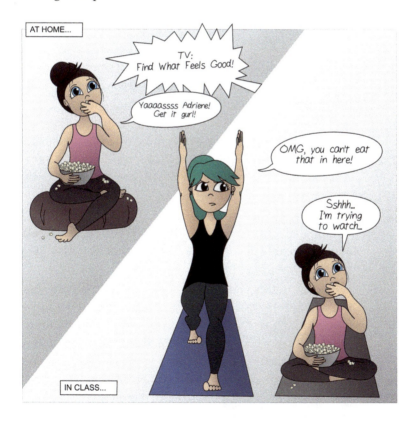

If the idea of paying for or attending classes turns you off when you know that you can practise yoga for free at home, consider the following:

- Many studios and clubs offer discounts on classes when paying for multiple sessions or month/year long memberships, which will encourage you to make it to all those classes so as to not have wasted your money.

- Compare the cost of a class to an indulgence of yours, such as that fancy latte, or drinks out at a restaurant or bar which really add up over time. You'll find some classes cost less than those indulgences and are better for you too!

- Invest in yourself! Your health and wellness are important and should be a priority. If classes are what it takes to build a solid practice, then go for it!

- You can meet new people with similar interests. In the age of social media, actually having a social life can be hard. And as an adult, don't even get me started on the challenges of making new friends!

- You might learn something new, which you take with you and incorporate in your home practice, and everyday life.

- Whatever results you are seeking from your practice, you will likely achieve quicker in a class setting. In the same way working out with a personal trainer can be more effective than going solo, so is practising yoga with an in-person instructor. Not only does a class setting provide mega motivation, your alignment, form and breathing will be kept in check by a teacher that is there to make sure you're doing it right.

- Classes allow you to escape real life if only for a little bit. It's like a mini vacation from work and home.

With that, you can take every precaution and measure to try to enjoy your class experience, and sometimes that just doesn't happen. It can be that another participant is not abiding by the too often unspoken code of ethics. It could be that you're not comfortable in a class setting. Or it could be the teacher.

Anybody can become a yoga teacher. Is your instructor a new or experienced teacher? One is not necessarily better for you than the other. An experienced teacher may have not attended another teacher's class in years, having become out of touch and stuck in their ways. Or they may be the funnest most knowledgeable teacher you'll ever meet. Maybe they've lost their passion. Or maybe, they've never been more eager. A new teacher can have decades of yoga experience under their belt, and then one day decided they were ready to pass on their knowledge. Or that new teacher might also be new to yoga, having taken one class and thought, hey I should teach this! A new teacher may lack variety in their sequences and pause awkwardly when trying to remember the next pose. Or maybe that new teacher stayed up for hours the night before prepping a meaningful and thoughtful class.

Your yoga instructor is *human*. It's important to remember that people can have a bad day and while your instructor should be doing what they can to ensure you have a good experience, they have off days too. Just like you.

So if you don't enjoy a class and think it may be because of the teacher, consider giving them a second chance. They're probably trying their best. Whatever you do, don't let it turn you away from your practice. Try a different class, with a different teacher. It's OK, teachers know that not everyone will like them. They'll be fine.

Home Practice

If you prefer to begin with a home practice, boy do you have a lot of options! With a home practice you are not restricted by the schedules offered by your local studios and clubs. All this freedom can make a home practice a little challenging to get going.

So where do you start? You can pick up a book that interests you, or find a video that suits your mood or needs.

Where books and videos differ is that while many books contain loads of wonderful information and amazing sequences to practise, for the beginner it can be frustrating to stop to turn a page between poses. What am I saying? That can be frustrating for anyone! However, don't knock it till you try it. Yoga books can be an amazing resource and there are so many on the market that you're sure to find something you love.

Videos, on the other hand, allow you to become completely absorbed in your practice by listening to the teacher's instructions while only occasionally having to look at the screen for clarification (just like in a class). Videos can be purchased in disc format, or online as downloads or streams. YouTube is a fantastic resource for free yoga classes. All you've got to do is search what you have in mind. If you draw a blank, here are some ideas of searches that will get you plenty of results: beginners yoga, yoga for back pain, yoga for weight loss, yoga for flexibility, yoga for strength, yoga for men. I could go on.

While a home practice is valuable and beneficial, it does have some pros and cons.

Pros

- If you need a pee break, you can pause your workout and go to the bathroom without disrupting a class.

- You can practise at any time of the day to suit your schedule.

- You can choose a routine that suits how you're feeling that day (tired, strong, back pain, etc.).

- You can pause a video or stay on the same page of a book to hold a particularly good pose a bit longer, without a class instructor moving you along before you want to.

- You can rewind a video or go back to your book if something is confusing and you need a little more time with it.

- With time you can develop your own routines, building confidence in your practice.

- You may have fewer distractions at home than at a club or studio.

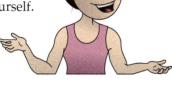

It's not that I'm not a people person, I just really don't like people...

- You don't have to leave the house.

- It's quality time for yourself.

- You can wear whatever the hell you want.

- It's free.

Cons

- If you lack motivation, it's easy to skip a workout/practice.

- If you get bored during a routine, you risk cutting it short.

- If your form is incorrect, there's no instructor there to correct you.

- If you are attempting advanced postures and doing them incorrectly, you can injure yourself.

- Unless you take the proper precautions, there can be tons of distractions at home: phone calls, texts, kids, Amazon packages at the door, etc.

- You might end up just sitting on your mat watching a video instead of participating.

- You don't get to potentially meet your new best yoga friend.

- You can't take advantage of the free equipment you can use at the studio/club (blocks, straps, etc.).

- If you spent $$$ on some kickass yoga gear, nobody will see it if you don't wear it out!

- If you have a question that's specific and hard to google, who are you gonna ask? Yell at the lady on the TV all you want, I can tell you from experience she isn't going to answer you.

So which one is better for you? A home or a class practice? Both have pros and cons that go beyond what I've already mentioned. So giving both a try is really the best way to decide.

Do both.

Read that again.

Do both.

While you might end up favouring one type of practice over the other, combining in-class and home practice is the best way to get the ultimate yoga experience. Aside from combining each one's positive aspects, here are some benefits to a well-rounded practice:

- An instructor's alignment tips and adjustments from class can be of great benefit for you at home.

- You can ask an instructor questions about something you practised at home and they'll be happy to help you.

- If you have to miss a class for whatever reason (scheduling conflict, a cold, etc.) having a home practice can help to make up for it.

- You can supplement a class practice by working on specific things at home that aren't the focus of the class, like split prep, deepening your backbend or getting your legs into lotus!

- If the classes you attend only put focus on asanas, you can practise the other limbs and branches at home on your own.

- If you want to take a break from classes, you don't have to lose all of your progress and hard work. Keep it up at home.

This isn't to say you need to regularly attend a class, dishing out more $$ than you want to. Showing up to a class here and there, trying new studios and clubs, different types of classes and styles of yoga can introduce you to something you can incorporate into your home practice. Maybe you'll want to sign up for a weekly class, or get an unlimited studio pass. You won't know until you try it.

FIVE

Where to Start?

There are so many different styles of yoga, some more traditional and well defined, some with a little more freedom of expression, it can be hard to know where to start.

Now that you've been bitten by the yoga bug, it's time to explore some of the styles you can try!

AcroYoga: The focus of AcroYoga is strength, flexibility and technique. AcroYoga combines yoga asana and acrobatics. It is usually practised in a group of three: a base (the stable one with the most contact to the ground), a flyer (the one who will be elevated or balanced with the assistance of the base) and a spotter (the one who stands next to the other two ready to catch the flyer if they slip or fall). This style helps to develop trust and communication. Maybe a little scary for a newbie, but not impossible. There are poses for all levels.

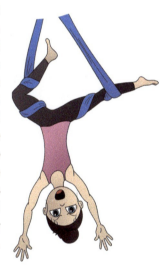

Aerial Yoga: a.k.a. Anti-Gravity Yoga. In aerial yoga a large silk hammock is suspended from the ceiling, strong enough to support the body. The silk allows you to perform poses mid-air and is supportive in backbends, forward folds and inversions. You can feel like an acrobat without the need to touch other people (like in AcroYoga)! This style of yoga is fairly new, so not much research has been conducted to prove it is more or less beneficial than another style. However, if you're feeling confident or want to spice things up a bit, why not give it a try? Check with the studio for any dress code related to this class: no jewelry, a top that covers your armpits, etc.

Ananda Yoga®: If you're looking for a safe and spiritual practice, Ananda Yoga offers yoga philosophy paired with asanas (poses), pranayama (breathing techniques) and meditation techniques. The poses in this style are suited to the practitioner and not the other way around. Meaning a pose will be modified or varied so that a yogi can do it, rather than trying to twist and pry a yogi's limbs to effect a posture that goes beyond their limits. As a result, you should never be out of breath in an Ananda class. It is not an aerobic style, it is relaxed. As your abilities develop and improve, the intensity of the poses you practise will increase to match. In Ananda Yoga, each asana is paired with an affirmation as you turn your focus inwards, striving to reach a higher consciousness.

Anusara Yoga: Anusara: "go with the flow" or "follow your heart". The goal of this style is to leave feeling joyful and empowered and to be able to bring those feelings outside of the class and into your everyday life. Anusara Yoga combines philosophies from Tantra Yoga with a series of over 250 poses and its own trademarked set of "Universal Alignment Principles". While there are no specific sequences of poses to practise in order, in an Anusara class, the teacher will guide you through a flow of core poses, encouraging variations to advance the poses or modifications where needed, then end the class in relaxation or meditation.

Ashtanga Yoga: A very common style of yoga practised all over the world, Ashtanga Yoga is a modern take on traditional yoga, founded by K. Pattabhi Jois in the 20th century. It focuses on the Eight Limbs of Yoga as described by Patanjali, and in particular, the first and second limbs (the yamas and the niyamas) and the third and fourth limbs (asanas and pranayama). Ashtanga is a vigorous style which serves to light an internal fire meant to purify the body. That means, you'll be working up a sweat. The practice of Ashtanga consists of several vinyasas (flows), typically beginning with several repetitions of Sun Salutations. Breath plays an important role in this style, as it syncs up with each pose you do. There are fundamental positions, a primary series, intermediate series and advanced series, all containing poses to be practised with consistency. It is not until you've mastered the poses in a series that you may move on to the next.

Baptiste Yoga™: Founded in the 1940s by Walt Baptiste, the Baptiste school of yoga is a Vinyasa style flow inspired by the teaching of B.K.S. Iyengar. Empowerment, strength and confidence are at the heart of this style. Instructors are specially trained in the Baptiste Methodology™ which boasts quality in their work, quick results, a down-to-earth approach to the practice and improved quality of life. Studios and retreats are located mainly in the US so unless you're in the area, you're more likely to practise this style with a video or book at home. Baron Baptiste, the son of Walt Baptiste has books and videos available online (including YouTube) and in stores. He is the founder of the Baptiste Institute (which conducts teacher training and host retreats, among other things) and the Baptiste Foundation. Classes include meditation and asana, they also include power and hot yoga elements.

Bikram Yoga: Designed by Bikram Choudhury in the 1970s, Bikram yoga is the style that popularized hot yoga, with temperatures in class being anywhere from 35°C to 42°C (95°F to 108°F). Many confuse hot yoga with Bikram yoga and vice versa. The difference between the styles is that Bikram Yoga can only be taught by Bikram certified teachers. Bikram Yoga is not just a style, it's an organization with roughly 700 franchises worldwide. In this style, there is a specific set of 26 postures (to begin) which are taught during a 90-minute class. The guidelines of Bikram yoga are strict and have often been questioned. However this style is safe to practise so long as you are properly hydrated and not performing postures beyond your means. In recent years, Bikram Choudhury himself has been surrounded by controversy as a result of multiple sexual misconduct and discrimination allegations. In 2016, a Los Angeles court stripped Choudhury of his beloved empire and awarded the whole shebang to the head of Bikram Yoga's legal team, and his main accuser, Minakshi Jafa-Bodden. In the midst of his legal troubles, and having denied all allegations against him, Choudhury fled to India. The company is currently being run by Miss Jafa-Bodden and continues to thrive under her rule, while we wait to see what happens with Choudhury...yikes!

Broga® Yoga: If you're a dude, this is something you've got to try. Broga®, through their various Brograms®, combines yoga with functional fitness for a unique experience geared towards men, working you inside and out. Its goal is to encourage more men to do yoga worldwide and to make sure they enjoy it.

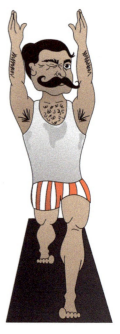

Hatha Yoga: This may be confusing, as you now know that Hatha Yoga simply means yoga postures. Therefore, any style of yoga where postures are practised can be called Hatha Yoga. True. However, many studios and clubs offer a class called Hatha Yoga. And you guessed it, it's a class focusing on yoga poses. Since the purpose of asanas in yoga is to prepare the body for breathing exercises, leading to meditation, those get incorporated into a Hatha class too. In a Hatha Yoga class, your teacher may design a class with any variety of the thousands of yoga poses out there, but will usually stick to the basics. Think of it as a sort of general class where the focus of the class may shift from week to week. This is a great class for beginners, as it may incorporate a bit of everything, including some flows through a series or postures and sometimes holding a pose for a longer amount of time. While in their teacher training, your instructor may learn a specific guideline for this type of class (for example supine postures, to seated postures, to standing postures, etc.), they may stray from that from time to time and have a little fun. Since its definition is broad, you should check out the site of the studio or club to see if their Hatha Yoga class is right for you.

Hot Yoga: Yoga that is hot. Set around temperatures of around 35°C to 42°C (95°F to 108°F), get ready to sweat! Hot Yoga differs from Bikram Yoga in that the instructors deviate from Bikram's strict set of postures and are not necessarily trained by the Bikram organization (although they could be I guess, if they trained there then wanted to do their own hot thing). The duration of the class may also vary from that 90-minute Bikram staple. Be sure to hydrate, and dress for the tropics. Before attending a class, you may want to check that your mat won't slip when wet. There are mats meant for Hot Yoga, and also towels you can apply over your mat to increase traction.

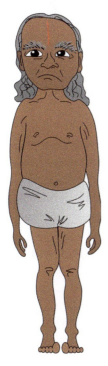

Iyengar Yoga: Based on the teachings developed in the 20th century by B.K.S. Iyengar, this style of yoga focuses strongly on proper alignment. Poses are typically held longer than usual and breath control is practised. Known to be therapeutic, everyone can practise this style as postural precision is encouraged with lots of modifications with the help of props: blocks, chairs, blankets, straps, etc.

Jivamukti Yoga: With a strong focus on Patanjali's interpretation of Asana, this style encourages compassion. In Jivamukti Yoga you will follow five tenets: Ahimsa (non-violence, compassion), Bhakti (devotion to a higher being, self-realization), Dhyana (meditation), Nada (union through sound) and Shastra (study, knowledge). A variety of classes are offered from Fundamentals to Open Class where proper alignment and safety in postures bring the practice together. Teachings involve the importance of one's relationship to other beings coming from a consistent place of joy. Their philosophy emphasizes the ethical treatment of animals, therefore vegetarianism/veganism is strongly encouraged.

Kundalini Yoga: Kundalini translates to "coiled one", which in yoga refers to the Shakti (energy source) located at the base of the spine. The spine in this style is likened to a serpent, rising from this coil, awakening the seven Chakras that begin at the base of the spine and work their way up to the crown of the head. Kundalini Yoga combines Bhakti Yoga (devotion and chanting), Raja Yoga (yoga of the mind), Tantra Yoga (expansion, awakening) and Asana (postures). The purpose of this style is to leave the practitioner with a sense of exuberance, increased awareness and higher consciousness by awakening subtle energies throughout the body, through movement, breathing techniques, meditation, visualization and chanting. Lots of chanting. And a gong! In a traditional Kundalini class, the practitioner avoids distraction that colour brings by wearing all white. Check with your local studio/club to see if this is recommended in their classes.

Kripalu Yoga: Listen to your body. That is what Kripalu Yoga teaches us. Founded in the 1980s by Amrit Desai, the style was named by Mr. Desai after his yoga teacher in India. In Hindu, kripalu means compassion. In Kripalu Yoga, we are gentle and compassionate towards ourselves. As with many other styles, you will find here a combination of asanas, breathing techniques and meditation. This style focuses strongly on the body. The challenge in this style comes from holding poses for a lot longer than other styles. You may also stay in meditation for quite some time as you focus on connecting to your inner self. Classes are often fun and playful. In this style, we practise safe poses with great care. It is suitable to all levels of practitioners.

Partner Yoga: While this style may be practised with a romantic partner, it does not have to be. Take a friend, a relative, a co-worker (or someone whose hands you're not afraid to hold). Traditional poses are transformed in this style so that they can be done together. Both partners will be holding a pose at all times so you're not taking turns, but doing things together. While some poses become more enjoyable to do with the support of your partner, others may become more challenging. Classes may be geared to couples for a date type session, others will be for everyone. In a class geared to couples, you can expect a lot of hand-holding and gazing into each other's eyes (so if you tend to giggle easily, prepare yourself!). In a regular class, you will still be expected to hold on to your partner or place your hands on them in some way so make sure you are comfortable with that. While size difference is not a major issue for most poses, it may affect some, but not so much that you shouldn't try it anyway! Partner Yoga is a great experience and a fun way to introduce a friend or loved one to yoga all while improving trust, self-awareness, communication and even your relationship.

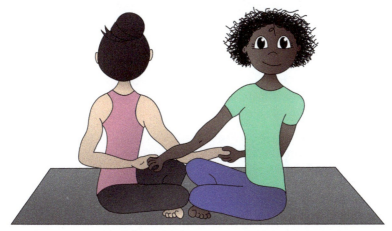

Power Yoga: Get ready for a good workout and get ready to sweat. In a Power Yoga class, you will be guided through a vigorous flow of poses focusing on building up the body through strength, balance, stamina and flexibility. You will be encouraged to connect your breath to your movements. This is an intense fitness-based style that is great for stress relief. Classes are typically fast paced and leave you feeling energized. Teachers can take many liberties in a Power Yoga class so classes may vary in temperature (there are Hot Power Yoga classes) and posture sequencing. Power Yoga is a style that was derived from Ashtanga sequencing by two American yogis who studied directly under Ashtanga's founder. Their goal was to make the strict style they learned more appealing and accessible to westerners and so, Power Yoga was born.

Prenatal Yoga: Prenatal Yoga classes are very beneficial to the expectant mother. Poses, breathing techniques, relaxation and meditation are all practised safely with your ever-changing body in mind. These practices are geared towards preparing your body for labour, to ease delivery and to benefit your journey along the way. What you practise in a prenatal class can help to alleviate many of the symptoms associated with pregnancy such as nausea, back pain, insomnia, stress, anxiety, etc. As your body changes through pregnancy, the relaxin hormone sets in and makes your joints all wonky, plus the weight of the baby weighs heavily on your bones and organs so there are some changes to your regular practice that need to be made. While you can attend any old yoga class you want while pregnant, it's best to take some precautions to make sure that you have a safe experience. If you're taking a general class, make sure that your teacher and you know which poses you should avoid and what modifications to make for other poses. Taking up a new exercise regime may not be advised for you during your pregnancy, so make sure if you are attending classes with higher intensity that it is something you were used to before you got knocked up. And as always, consult with your doctor before taking up any kind of activity while pregnant.

Restorative Yoga: Based heavily on the teachings of B.K.S. Iyengar with its encouraged use of props, Restorative Yoga is meant to restore balance to the body, mind and spirit. In a typical class, you will practise deep breathing and just a small handful of poses compared to other styles. These poses are safe and modified as needed with the use of props and are held for very long periods of time, sometimes up to five minutes. This class should be relaxing and recuperative, perfect if you are recovering from an injury, need to de-stress or unwind, are hungover, are on a rest day, or L ' 'are just in need of some healing. It goes without saying that this class is suitable for everyone.

Sivananda Yoga: Sivananda is a holistic approach to yoga that encourages lots of relaxation and focuses on deep breathing techniques, diet, positive thinking, meditation and postures to promote flexibility and toned muscles, leading to a healthy body, inside and out. In Sivananda Yoga vegetarianism is encouraged. An Ayurvedic (see chapters 6 and 14) diet is followed, consuming sattvic foods and avoiding rajasic and tamasic foods to give the body the positive energy needed to achieve optimum health. A typical class may begin in Savasana (Corpse Pose), then include some breathing techniques, a few Sun Salutations, followed by Sivananda's 12 basic asanas and ending in deep relaxation. The atmosphere of a Sivananda class is pleasant and relaxed with a slow pace, perfect for everyone. Variations of the postures may be taken based on the level of the practitioner, with relaxation poses following each posture throughout the class.

Tantra Yoga: We already know that the purpose of Tantra Yoga is to achieve bliss. So what would we do as part of a Tantra Yoga practice? Well, this style can be practised alone or with a partner. It is a very intimate practice that deepens your connection to yourself and to others, increases your self-awareness, improves your confidence and emotional balance and promotes happiness, or bliss, in both our conscious and subconscious states. So aside from practising postures, breathing techniques and meditation, in Tantra Yoga other rituals are explored such as mantras, mudras (locks), visualization, and spiritual and physical cleansing. Yes, intestinal cleansing is encouraged. The hippies in the 60s and 70s popularized Tantra Yoga with Tantric sex, which promotes certain positions to improve your sex life. It's important to remember that while this is one benefit of this practice, there is a lot more to Tantra Yoga than sex. In its origin, Tantra Yoga sought to understand the differences and to find balance between the two Hindu deities Shakti and Shiva, representing the male and female dynamics of the universe. Complex, right?

Vinyasa Yoga: A vinyasa refers to a flow, movement or sequence of yoga postures, strung together and paired with regulated breathing that follows your movements. In this sense, any yoga class where postures are practised in a flowy sequence can be called a Vinyasa Yoga class. Smaller groups of sequences such as Sun Salutations or the Ashtanga series can be strung together to make up a full class. So by definition, Ashtanga Yoga is a type of Vinyasa Yoga (but with its own set of guidelines and practices) as are many other styles. The idea is to flow seamlessly, dynamically, from one pose to the next. This is a very popular style of yoga that is typically a little more fast paced than a Hatha Yoga class (but less so than a Power Yoga class) where you're bound to work up a bit of a sweat and come out feeling reinvigorated. The constant change of position in a Vinyasa class keeps you alert and focused, improving your mental awareness and concentration. Calling a class Vinyasa Yoga means the instructor has the freedom and creativity to take you on the journey of their choosing, while still following the main principles and purposes of a yoga practice. You are sure to practise postures from multiple positions, working on balance, flexibility, strength and stamina, even incorporating some breathing exercises and relaxation.

Yin Yoga: Yin Yoga is a relaxed style of yoga with a slower pace in which poses are held for a long time, anywhere from 30-45 seconds for a beginner to upwards of five minutes for an advanced level student. As with all asana based practices, Yin Yoga is designed to prepare the body for long periods of sitting for meditation. Therefore, emphasis is put on increasing range of motion in the joints and flexibility in the muscles, especially through the knees and hips by getting deep into the fascia (or connective tissue). This style boasts many benefits such as helping to regulate energy levels, reducing stress and anxiety and improving circulation, flexibility and joint mobility.

Yoga for Kids: Yoga classes designed for children and teens differ from those for adults in that kids and teens have a harder time sitting still and being quiet (though some adults do too!) so they are not made to hold poses for very long. A kids' class is usually louder and more interactive. Some simple breathing techniques may be practised, but kids are not likely to follow specific or complicated breathing patterns throughout a sequence of poses so this is not enforced. Kids and teens also tend to be naturally more flexible than adults, so caution is taken in some poses to ensure that our little yogis do not go beyond a safe range of motion and hyperextend. They can get bored easily so these classes may be shorter depending on the age group, and have more of a fun vibe to them, sometimes involving music or games. There are many benefits that our younger counterparts can reap from a regular yoga practice. It can improve their concentration, confidence, sleep patterns, coordination, balance and strength. They will learn stress management and self-calming skills. Introducing yoga to kids and teens early on can provide them with valuable skills that they can take with them into adulthood.

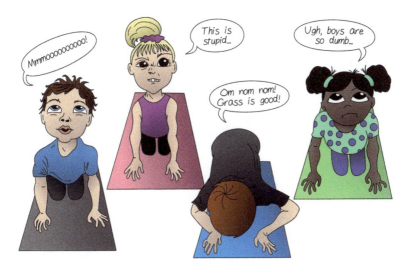

Yoga for Seniors: You're never too old to start a yoga practice, and yoga classes geared towards golden girls and boys are very inclusive to beginners. In this type of class, the instructor will keep aging bodies and their potential ailments and limits in mind. Generally a slower, safe and gentle practice is what you will experience with movements and breathing techniques geared towards your abilities. With yoga being low-impact, it's a great form of exercise for aging practitioners helping them to maintain and even improve their balance, strength, flexibility and stamina. Along with these physical health benefits, you will experience mental and emotional well-being helping you to feel healthier inside and out.

Woah. That's a lot of yoga.

Aside from the multitude of more classical yoga styles available to you, other, less traditional classes might include: Goat Yoga, Beer Yoga, Wine & Yoga, Angry Yoga, Naked Yoga...they are all what they sound like and more.

There exists as well workshops and retreats which are both worth considering once you've decided to dedicate yourself to your practice. Since these can be a little more costly and require somewhat of a commitment, it's prudent to start with something a little smaller.

Just as describing the taste of a food to someone who's never tried it just can't do it justice, it's important to experience a form of yoga to really understand it.

The variety of yoga schools out there can be overwhelming, and with studios and YouTubers coming up with clever names for their classes, it can be confusing. Yoga is ever evolving and complex. Instead of trying to "figure it out", "master it" or simply "keep up", consider yourself a student of the practice. As yogis, we will always have more to learn and experience. To do this, we must try new things.

SIX

Yoga Lingo

Yoga can sound a lot more complicated than it is. Because yoga is such an ancient practice, it is, of course, taught using an ancient language: Sanskrit.

Not every teacher will use Sanskrit words in their classes. They know that it's not likely that you know what they mean. Many teachers, however, will include a word or term here or there that you will familiarize yourself with over time. This will commonly be the name of an asana (see what I did there?), and the reason why instructors do this is not just to teach you these words, but to use them often enough so that they themselves don't forget what they mean!

Sanskrit is a beautiful language. Its words can be difficult to translate since many Sanskrit words have a vast, complex meaning. The earliest written form of Sanskrit that we know of dates back to at least 1500 BC, the Vedic age of ancient India. The Vedic knowledge contained in writings (which included yoga philosophy) was before then passed on orally, making Sanskrit one of the oldest languages in the world.

You have certainly heard some Sanskrit words before picking up this book (namaste, anyone?) and after just a few chapters, you are now becoming familiar with a few more. While many of these terms can't really be directly translated to just one word, we know that in yoga, they refer to a general idea or something more specific.

Anjali Mudra = a common mudra, where the hands are held together in prayer position
Anna Yoga = the yoga of food and nourishment

Asana = postures
Ayurveda = medical knowledge and philosophy passed down by the Vedics
Bandha = body locks
Bhakti = the yoga of devotion
Chakra = seven energy centres found within our bodies
Dharana = concentration
Dhyana = meditation
Drishti = a focused gaze (inward or outward)
Hatha Yoga = the physical practice of yoga
Jnana Yoga = the yoga of wisdom
Karma Yoga = the yoga of action
Malas = a set of beads used to count the repetition of a chant or mantra
Mantra = a sound, word or phrase that is repeated to aid in concentration
Mudra = a symbolic hand gesture
Nadi = energy channels within the body, weaving through the spinal cord and chakras
Namaste = a greeting meaning: The light in me bows to the light in you.
Niyamas = personal standards, self-discipline
Om = the most sacred of mantras chanted before and/or after many rituals/practices
Pranayama = breathing techniques
Pratyahara = sensory withdrawal
Raja Yoga = yoga of the mind
Sadhana = the discipline of practising yoga through asana, meditation, prayer, etc.
Samadhi = pure consciousness
Surya Namaskar = Sun Salutation

Sutra = (in yoga) a proverb, rule or belief in literature of yoga philosophy
Tantra Yoga = the yoga of awakening
Veda = ancient sacred writings composed in Sanskrit
Vinyasa = movement or flow or postures strung together
Yamas = ethical standards
Yoga = to join, to unite

Other Sanskrit terms you will become familiar with over time are the names for certain poses which we will explore next!

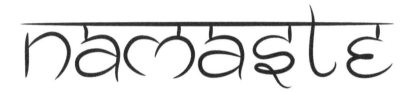

SEVEN

Strike a Pose!

Yoga poses are meant to prepare the body for long periods of sitting in meditation. The toning, strengthening, improved balance and increased flexibility and stamina are all a happy bonus to a consistent practice. Luckily, there are thousands of poses, variations and modifications for you to choose from. Variety is the spice of life. Switching up your yoga routine will keep your body guessing and keep you interested.

The poses listed here will get you started and are sure to give you the confidence to venture off and explore beyond.

Without the guidance of an in-person teacher, however, you may be unsure if you are doing a pose correctly, or if there is something you can do to make it better. Some tips that might help you include:

- Practise in front of a mirror: focus on the alignment cues provided.

- Listen to your body: if something hurts, don't do it.

- Do some research: if there is a pose that is particularly frustrating to you, find out more about it, look up tips, variations and modifications.

- Film yourself: set up your cell phone on selfie mode and take a video of yourself doing a sequence or series of poses so that you can act as an outsider looking in. You may gain some insight and be able to make some simple adjustments.

- Watch first, then do: if you're following a video, watch through it first, make sure you are comfortable with the practice you're about to take on, then do it. If you're following a sequence from a book, read through the poses and their descriptions first before starting.

When you are just starting out, your practice should not be complicated. Start with shorter sequences of simple poses that you understand and can do well. If you are getting out of breath, or needing to force your body into certain positions that cause you stress and pain, reel it in. The next time you practise, try something new, but make sure it's not overwhelming. Maybe add in one or two new poses to your routine every now and then to increase your repertoire. Don't allow yourself to get discouraged. Do poses, sequences, videos, etc. that you enjoy and find ways to make it fun. Practise at least three times a week and you'll be sure to see improvement. Remember: Practice makes progress!

Easy Pose (*Sukhasana*)

Sit cross-legged on your mat. Your legs should be crossed at the shins with your feet beneath the knees of the opposite legs. Criss-cross-applesauce. When you look down, you should see a triangle with your crotch and knee folds being the three points. Make sure that you are not tucking your pelvis back or rounding out your spine. Tilt your pelvis slightly forward without arching in the lower back. Lay your hands in your lap palms facing up, or on your knees, palms facing down. Sit up nice and tall with your shoulder blades drawn back and down, lifting through the chest. Your head should be aligned directly over your tailbone, chin parallel to the floor or slightly tucked down, elongating the back of the neck.

Variation/Modification: place a folded blanket or cushion beneath your tush to elevate tight hips and relieve tension in the knees.

Cautions: avoid this pose if your knees are messed up; if you sit this way often, remember to alternate which leg crosses over the other to even out your joints.

Benefits: helps to calm the mind and de-stress; strengthens the back and stretches out the knees and ankles; opens up the hips, groin and outer thighs.

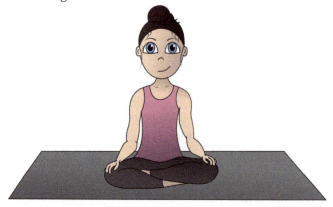

Mountain Pose (*Tadasana*)

Stand up tall with your feet together. If this is uncomfortable or makes it hard to hold your balance, step your feet hip width apart. Focus on your alignment and form from the bottom up. Distribute your weight evenly across all four corners of each foot (the ball under the big toe, the ball under the baby toe and either side of your heel). Stack your knees over your ankles, then your hips over your knees. Engage your quadriceps, rotating them slightly inward. Make sure that your pelvis is in a neutral position. Tighten up through your core, squeezing everything toward the centre of your body. Draw your shoulders down and back, lining them up over your hips. Stay long through the spine and neck, keeping your chin parallel to the mat, ears stacked over your shoulders. Keep your arms at your sides, rotated so that the palms are slightly turned out or bring your hands together in prayer position (Anjali Mudra) at chest height, thumbs resting on your sternum to remind you to keep your chest lifted. Breathe slowly and with control all the while imagining an upward lifting energy through the front of the body and a downward flowing, grounding energy through the back of the body. Hold for 30 seconds or longer.

Variation/Modification: challenge your balance by practising Mountain Pose with your eyes closed.

Cautions: avoid this pose if you're experiencing low blood pressure, headaches or dizziness.

Benefits: strengthens the legs, glutes and abdominals; improves posture and stability; can relieve back pain, sciatica and helps to relieve flat feet.

Upward Salute (*Urdhva Hastasana*)

From Mountain Pose, arms at your sides, palms slightly turned out, sweep your arms up overhead. Allow your arms to rotate naturally from the shoulders as they rise. Avoid popping the ribs out and lifting the shoulders. Stay long through the torso and keep a neutral pelvis. Bring the palms of your hands together overhead, starting at the base, working your way up to your fingertips. Reach through your pinkies, allowing your thumbs to point back and down towards you as you gaze up at them. Hold for 3-5 breaths. To release, on an exhale, lower your hands in prayer position to chest height. If you're following or creating a sequence, you can proceed directly to a Standing Forward Bend by sweeping your arms down as you fold forward from the hips.

Variation/Modification: alternatively, you can bring your hands together at chest height, then slowly and carefully raise them up to eye level, winging your elbows out to the sides as much as is comfortable for you (max winging = shoulder height), gazing at your thumbs. Another option: you can hold Mountain Pose with your hands in prayer position (Anjali Mudra).

Cautions: if you have shoulder pain, keep your arms parallel to each other overhead, palms facing in, instead of bringing your hands together. For shoulder injuries, avoid raising your arms up overhead altogether. For neck injuries, keep your gaze forward and avoid raising your arms up overhead. Avoid this pose if you are experiencing a headache, or dizziness.

Benefits: stretches the front torso, sides of the body and shoulders; strengthens the legs and glutes; improves stability and posture.

Cat Pose/Cow Pose (*Marjaryasana/Bitilasana*)

Begin in Table Pose (on all fours) with your wrists stacked under your shoulders and your knees stacked under your hips. Your feet should be about hip width apart with your toes facing straight back (not in towards each other). Spread your fingers wide, and press your fingertips into the mat to relieve tension in the wrists. Press down through the tops of your feet to relieve pressure from the knees. On an inhale, lower your belly towards the mat as you lift your chest and gaze up, staying long in the neck. This is Cow Pose. On your exhale, tuck your navel up towards your spine as you round your back up. This is Cat Pose. Throughout both poses, your head and neck should stay in line with your upper back (up in Cow, down in Cat). Continue alternating these poses following your breath, all the while staying firm through the fingertips, arms and tops of the feet. Repeat for 1-3 minutes.

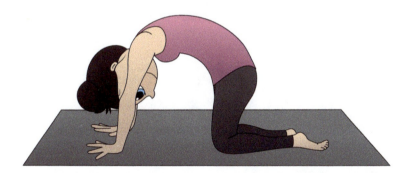

Variation/Modification: Cat/Cow Pose is an excellent warm up for your spine and stretch for your abdominals. Encourage oblique stretches by Wagging the Tail. Shift your hips from side to side as though you were...wagging a tail...looking over your right shoulder when you shift your hips to the right and vice versa. Continue to move with your breath. Once both of these movements become comfortable, combine Cat/Cow and Wagging the Tail so that you are making circular motions with your torso, allowing your breath to flow naturally.

Cat/Cow continued...

Cautions: if you have a back injury or are in your 2nd or 3rd trimester of pregnancy, proceed slowly and with caution, avoiding one pose or the other by alternating instead between Cow or Cat Pose and a neutral spine; if you have a wrist injury or pain, you can do this sequence on fists or drop to your forearms, or from Easy Pose; if you have bad knees, avoid staying in these poses for long.

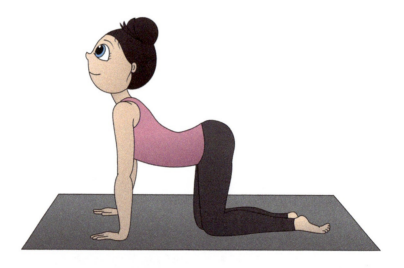

Benefits: stretches the abdominals, back, neck; strengthens the core and spine; increases flexibility in the spine; improves coordination; warms up the torso for more advanced poses; stimulates the abdominal organs; relieves stress; can relieve lower back pain and sciatica.

Downward Facing Dog (*Adho Mukha Svanasana*)

From Table Pose (all fours), line up your wrists under your shoulders and your knees under your hips. Spread your fingers out wide and press your fingertips into the mat. Curl your toes under and on an exhale, lift your knees up off the mat, reaching your tailbone up towards the sky and back. Meanwhile, press the front of your mat away from you with your hands, lengthening through the spine and stretching through the arms and shoulders. If your flexibility allows, touch your heels down to the mat. If not, do not force them, you may get there in time (you may not, and that's OK). Line your ears up with your arms, keeping your gaze back towards your feet, neck in line with your spine (no dangling heads!). Release on an exhale as you bend your knees, returning to Table Pose, or follow through another transition as instructed.

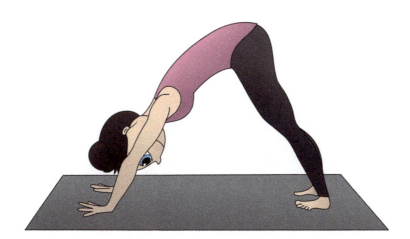

Down Dog continued...

Variation/Modification: Three Legged Dog - from Downward Facing Dog, raise your right leg up high. Your foot can be flexed or pointed. If flexed, reach through your heel. If pointed, reach through your toes. Try to keep your hips squared off to the mat as much as possible as you continue to press evenly through both hands. Release on an exhale and repeat with the other leg.

Cautions: avoid this pose if you have severe carpal tunnel syndrome, an ear infection or are in your 3rd trimester of pregnancy; if you have neck, shoulder and/or back injuries, be cautious and modify to Table Pose as needed.

Benefits: stretches the arches of the feet, hands, shoulders, and the entire back of the body; strengthens the arms, shoulders and legs; calms the mind; relieves stress, headaches and fatigue; improves digestion and symptoms of sciatica.

Standing Forward Fold (*Uttanasana*)

Begin in Mountain Pose with your hands at your sides or on your hips. (Alternatively you can get to Standing Forward Bend by stepping your feet up to a forward fold from Downward Facing Dog.) On your exhale, fold forward from the hips (not the waist), lowering your belly towards the tops of your thighs and keeping your back straight for as long as possible. Keep a slight bend in the knees to avoid locking them. Reach your fingertips or palms to the mat on either side of your feet. If your flexibility has yet to allow you to reach the floor, don't force it, instead, hug your elbows as you hold the pose with slightly bent knees. With each inhale, feel your spine getting longer and with each exhale, allow yourself to sink deeper into the fold. Allow your head to hang, keeping your neck in line with your spine without forcing it any which way. Hold for 3-5 breaths. To release, on an inhale, tighten up through the core as you bend deeper in the knees and raise your torso, straightening up to standing, with your arms at your sides or hands on your hips.

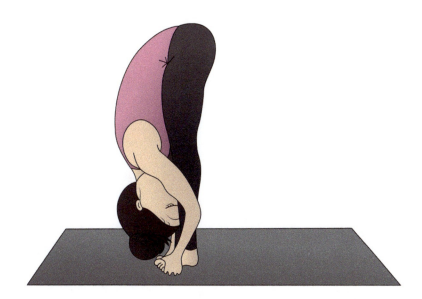

Forward Fold continued...

Variation/Modification: find more length through the spine by starting in Mountain Pose, and inhaling as you raise your arms up overhead to Upward Salute. Immediately on an exhale, go into your fold, reaching long through your fingertips as you sweep your arms down. To release, tighten up through your core, bend the knees slightly and on an inhale, raise your torso as you sweep your arms back up. With your arms overhead at the top of your inhale, exhale, bringing your palms together as you lower your hands to your heart in prayer position (Anjali Mudra).

Cautions: if you have a back injury, keep your knees bent as deeply as needed to perform this pose or place a block under your hands to bring the floor closer to you.

Benefits: stretches the hips and the back of your legs; increases flexibility in the hamstrings and calves; releases the neck and shoulders; improves digestion; reduces stress, anxiety and fatigue.

Standing Half Forward Fold (*Ardha Uttanasana*)

Start from a Standing Forward Bend. If in this pose your hands are touching down to the mat, come up onto your fingertips with your hands slightly in front of your feet. If you're hugging your elbows, gently place your hands on your shins. Keep a slight bend in your knees and avoid locking them back. On your next inhale, lift your chest up and away from your legs and straighten out your back as much as you can. Your neck should stay in line with your spine and your gaze should be slightly forward or down towards your mat. With your fingertips down, press into the mat to help you in the lift. If your back stays rounded, place your hands on your shins as high as you need to straighten out your torso. Hold for 3-5 breaths then release on an exhale by returning to Standing Forward Bend.

Variation/Modification: if you're having a hard time straightening out your back, or even if it's just more comfortable for you, place your hands either on the tops of your thighs, on blocks, on the back of a chair, or up against a wall, instead of on your shins/mat.

Cautions: if you have a back injury or are in your 2nd or 3rd trimester of pregnancy, widen your stance and bend your knees as much as necessary to feel stable and comfortable; if you're a sciatica sufferer, widen your stance and turn your toes slightly inward; if you have neck issues, keep your head low and avoid gazing forward.

Benefits: stretches the hips, the back of your legs and front torso; increases flexibility in the hamstrings and calves; strengthens the back; improves your posture.

Chair Pose (*Utkatasana*)

Standing in Mountain Pose, raise your arms up overhead (palms together or shoulder width apart, palms facing in). On your exhale, bend at the knees, keeping them together and even with each other, sending your tush back and lowering it until your thighs are as parallel to the mat as possible. Keep your chest lifted and your chin up. Put a little weight in your heels and stay connected to the balls under your big toes and baby toes. While shifting your weight back, connect to your hamstrings and glutes, and tighten up your core. Keep your shoulder blades down and back as you lengthen through the spine. Focus on keeping the knees stacked above the ankles as much as possible. Hold for 3-5 breaths. Exhale as you return to standing with your arms down at your sides or in prayer position at chest height. Alternatively, you may hold this posture with feet hip width apart, adding engagement to the inner thigh muscles.

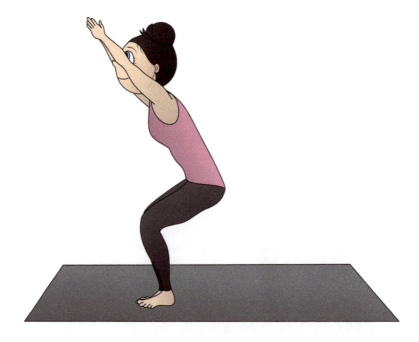

Chair Pose continued...

Variation/Modification: place a rolled-up towel or mat under your heels, this will ease tension in the ankles and other joints; try this pose with your back up against the wall, lowering your hips to be in line with your knees or slightly higher (never lower) and stacking your knees over your ankles (gym class, anyone?).

Caution: if you have a knee injury, lower slowly and proceed with caution, try not to let your knees pass your ankles; if you have a shoulder injury and cannot bring your arms up overhead, or if you have high blood pressure, bring the palms of your hands together in Anjali Mudra (prayer position) at chest height.

Benefits: strengthens the ankles, calves, legs, back and hip flexors; opens the chest and shoulder girdles; helps to relieve flat feet.

Garland Pose (*Malasana*)

From Mountain Pose, step your feet out to about shoulder width apart, toes slightly turned out. Bend your knees as you lower your hips to a deep, low squat. Widen your knees so that your torso fits between them. Keep your chest lifted and stay long through the back and neck. Keep your heels connected to the mat if you can (otherwise, keep them slightly lifted). Shift your feet to find a comfortable position. (You want your feet to be as close together as possible while keeping your heels low and knees wide apart.) Press your elbows and upper arms up against your knees to open up the hips as you bring your hands together in prayer position (Anjali Mudra) with your thumbs resting on your sternum. At the same time, engage your legs, squeezing them back in towards your arms. Breathe deeply, holding Garland Pose for three breaths or longer.

Variation/Modification: if your heels don't touch down and keeping them lifted is giving you charley horses, place a blanket or rolled-up mat beneath them. If this pose is easy, start practising it with your feet closer and closer together.

Cautions: avoid this pose if you have a recent knee or lower back injury.

Benefits: stretches the ankles, thighs, groin and hips; strengthens the abdominals; improves balance and focus; can help to prepare the pregnant yogi for childbirth.

Tree Pose (*Vrksasana*)

Standing in Mountain Pose with your arms at your sides, shift your weight to your left foot. Bend the right knee and bring the sole of your right foot to the inside of your left leg in one of three positions: 1- up against your lower calf/ankle with your toes resting down on the mat; 2- against your calf just below the knee; 3- against your inner thigh, by grabbing your right ankle with your right hand to get yourself there. Avoid placing your foot on the knee joint. Press your right foot into your left leg and your left leg back into your right foot with equal pressure, bringing all your energy to the centre line. Tighten up the muscles in your grounded leg, glutes and core and open up the right side hip. Bring your hands to prayer position at chest height, thumbs resting on your sternum to remind you to keep your chest lifted (Anjali Mudra). Find a focal point that isn't moving and slow down your breath. Option: inhale and lift your arms up and overhead, reaching through the fingertips, palms facing in towards each other. If your shoulders allow, you can bring your hands to prayer position overhead. Hold for 3-5 breaths, then repeat on the other side.

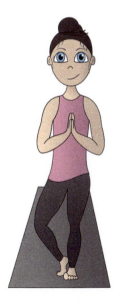
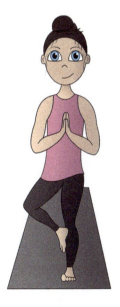
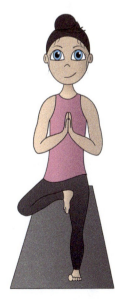

Tree Pose continued...

Variation/Modification: if you are having trouble balancing, use a wall for support by placing the hand of the same side as the grounded foot on the wall, and bringing your opposite hand to half prayer position at chest height, or overhead.

Cautions: if you have high blood pressure, avoid raising your arms up overhead; if you have an existing ankle injury, avoid balancing on the affected leg.

Benefits: strengthens the ankles, calves, thighs and spine; stretches the inner thighs, groin, chest and shoulders; improves balance; relieves sciatica; helps to relieve flat feet.

Warrior I (*Virabhadrasana I*)

From Mountain Pose, step your right leg back, connecting your right heel to the mat with the toes slightly turned out. Press that right foot firmly into the mat and remain engaged throughout the right leg. Bend the left leg, stacking the knee above the ankle joint (never passing it). Make sure your knee is pointing straight ahead in the same direction as your toes (not in or out). If this is easy and you want to lower your body further, widen your stance so that you can keep your left knee over your ankle by stepping your right leg back a bit further. Square your shoulders off towards the front short edge of your mat, and encourage your hips to follow suit as much as possible, without forcing them. Keep your core engaged as you lengthen through the spine. Raise your arms up overhead, palms together or shoulder width apart with your palms facing in. Spread your shoulder blades wide, stay long through the neck and bring your gaze either straight ahead or up towards your hands. Alternatively, you can bring your hands to prayer position (Anjali Mudra) at chest height and gaze forward. Hold for 3-5 breaths on each side (unless you're following or creating a sequence that directs you otherwise).

Variation/Modification: bring your arms to cactus position: out wide to either side with your upper arms parallel to the floor, elbows bent at 90°, palms facing forward. Lean the torso back gently, lifting the chest and gazing slightly up. This is a great chest opener if you feel tight in that area or if you sit at a computer or desk for long periods of time.

Cautions: if you have a shoulder injury, keep your arms low, or if raising overhead, keep your arms parallel to each other, palms not touching; if you have neck issues, avoid gazing up by keeping your head in a neutral position; for ankle injuries/reduced range of motion in the ankles, keep your back heel lifted.

Warrior I continued…

Benefits: strengthens your shoulders, arms, legs, ankles and back; stretches the arms, legs, shoulders, abdominals and groin; improves balance.

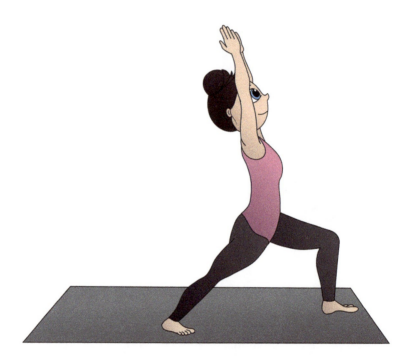

Warrior II (*Virabhadrasana II*)

From Mountain Pose, facing the short edge of your mat, step your right foot back, turning it out to a 90° angle, keeping your left toes facing forward. Alternatively, you may start in a wide stance facing the long edge of your mat, and rotating your left foot out to face the short edge of your mat. With your torso facing the long edge of your mat, bring your arms out to either side at shoulder level, parallel to the floor, palms facing down. Keep your right leg straight (without locking the knee) and bend your left leg so that your knee is stacked above your ankle, without passing it. If you want to lower your body further, widen your stance instead of bending more in the left knee so that you maintain proper stacking of the joints in your left leg. Make sure your left knee is facing the same direction as your toes (not leaning in or out). Your hips should be level with each other, so if your right hip is much higher than the left, adjust your stance to even them out. Maintain a neutral pelvis (don't stick your butt out), lengthen out through the spine and the neck and keep your shoulders down and back, away from your ears. Tighten up through the core and stay strong in the shoulders and arms. Actively reach through both hands, gazing over the middle finger of your left hand. Hold for 3-5 breaths, then repeat on the other side.

Variation/Modification: transition to Humble Warrior: keeping your legs firmly in Warrior II position, interlace your fingers behind your back then fold forward from the hips, lowering your torso to the inside of your bent knee as you raise your arms up towards the ceiling.

Cautions: for neck injuries, avoid turning your head to look over your front hand; for severe shoulder injuries, keep your hands on your hips or in prayer position at chest height.

Warrior II continued...

Benefits: strengthens the legs and ankles; stretches the hips, legs, ankles, shoulders and chest; improves balance, concentration and circulation; increases stamina; helps to relieve flat feet and sciatica.

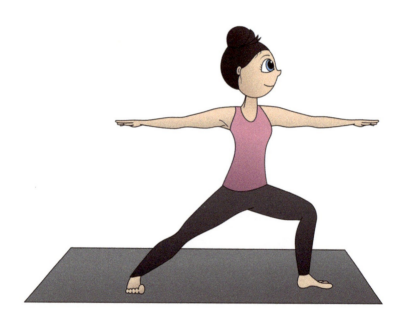

Triangle (*Trikonasana*)

From Mountain Pose, step your right foot back, turning it out to a 90° angle, keeping your left toes facing forward and keeping both legs straight without locking the knees. Alternatively, you may start in a wide stance facing the long edge of your mat, and rotating your left foot out to face the short edge of your mat. You can also get here from Warrior II by simply straightening out your bent leg. With your torso facing the long edge of your mat, raise your arms out to your sides, shoulder level, parallel to the floor, palms facing down. Shift your hips to the right as you slide your torso to the left, reaching long through the left hand. Bend sideways to the left, placing the back of your left hand against your inner, lower left leg (or grab onto your left shin), while the right arm reaches up towards the ceiling. Stay strong through the legs, keeping the chest wide and open. Gaze straight ahead or up towards your right hand. Hold for 3-5 breaths, then repeat on the other side.

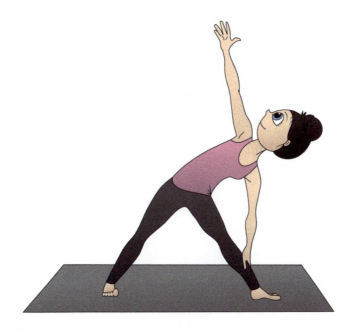

Triangle continued...

Variation/Modification: if you feel unsteady in Triangle Pose, stagger your feet so that they are not lined up like on a tightrope, but hip width apart, like on train tracks. If your left foot is forward, place it nearer the top left corner of your mat while your right foot is near the back right corner. You can also use a yoga block for support by placing it at the top of your mat in line with your back foot to hold onto instead of resting your hand against your leg.

Cautions: if you have a neck injury, keep your gaze ahead of you or down at the mat (not up); for shoulder injuries, bring the arm extending up to rest on your side, or gently bind it behind your back.

Benefits: engages the whole body; stretches the hamstrings, groin, hips, chest and shoulders; strengthens the thighs, hips and back; improves balance and concentration; helps to relieve lower back pain, symptoms of flat feet and sciatica.

Low Lunge (*Anjaneyasana*)

There are a few ways to get into a Low Lunge. One would be from Downward Facing Dog. Step your left foot forward between your hands. Another is from a Standing Forward Bend. Bend your knees as needed to place your palms down on either side of your feet, then step your right foot back. You can also get there from Triangle Pose or Warrior I or II. Start by rotating your back foot forward as you lower your torso, bringing your hands down on either side of your front foot. However you decide to get there, once you have your feet apart as described in the examples above, check to make sure they are not lined up one behind the other (like on a tightrope) but staggered to be hip width apart. Your front knee should be stacked over your front ankle, facing the same direction as your toes. Lower your back knee to the mat, followed by the top of your foot. Put some pressure into the top of your back foot to relieve some tension from the knee. Tighten up through the legs and core. On an inhale, raise your torso, arms up overhead parallel to each other, palms facing in. Gaze forward or up towards your hands. On your exhales, relax into the hips. Hold for 3-5 breaths. To release, lower your hands to the mat on either side of your front foot, curl the toes of your back foot under and lift the knee. From here you can slide your front foot back to Downward Facing Dog or Plank Pose, or you can shift the hips up and slide the back foot up to a Standing Forward Bend. Repeat on the other side.

Variation/Modification: if it's difficult to raise your arms up, you can keep your fingertips down on either side of your front leg, place your hands on your hips, or hold Anjali Mudra (prayer position) at heart level. If getting your arms up is an issue of balance vs injury, you can work your way there by first propping your arms up onto your front thigh and slowly raising them overhead, one at a time or together.

Low Lunge continued...

Cautions: for knee injuries, place a blanket or folded-up mat under your grounded knee and be cautious with the position of your front knee, leaning against a wall for extra stability; avoid this pose if you have heart problems or high blood pressure.

Benefits: stretches the thighs and hips; strengthens the legs, back and shoulders; improves balance; opens the chest.

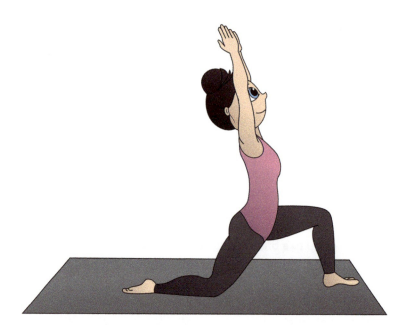

Plank Pose (*Phalakasana*)

From Table Pose, align your wrists under your shoulders and spread your fingers wide while pressing your fingertips into the mat. Engage tightly through your core as you send one leg straight back followed by the other, resting on the balls of your toes and reaching back through your heels. Stay strong in the shoulders and legs. Keep your hips low without dipping in the lower back. Your body should form a straight line from your shoulders to your ankles, if not slightly rounded at the shoulder blades. Take your gaze down towards the mat, keeping your neck in line with your spine (without dropping the head). Hold for 3-5 controlled breaths. To release, gently lower your knees and return to Table Pose or push back to Child's Pose (it's coming up, you'll love it).

Variation/Modification: if you are having a hard time holding a full plank for longer than a full breath, hold for as long as you can, then gently bring your knees down to the mat, keeping your hips low and maintaining a straight line from your head to your knees for the duration of the pose.

Cautions: if you have severe carpal tunnel syndrome, modify this pose by forming fists with your hands, or by lowering onto your forearms; for lower back injuries, gently lower to your knees.

Benefits: strengthens the arms, chest, wrists, lower back and core muscles; improves posture; builds endurance.

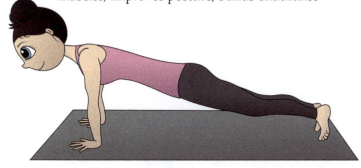

Sphinx Pose (*Salamba Bhujangasana*)

Start by lying face-down on your mat, feet hip width apart. Lift your chest, bringing your forearms parallel to each other on the mat, elbows stacked directly beneath your shoulders. Press through your forearms to gain length through your spine as you lift through your front torso, coming to a gentle, low backbend. Lengthen through your neck, keeping your gaze forward. Reach your tailbone back as you let your pelvis sink into the mat. Keep your leg muscles engaged without flexing and reach through your toes. Make sure that your toes are facing straight back and not in towards each other. Breathe steadily and with control. Hold for 5-10 breaths, then lower the chest to release.

Variation/Modification: for a challenging core exercise, alternate between Sphinx Pose and Dolphin Plank (a forearm plank). Hold Sphinx Pose for three full breaths, then slowly and with control, keeping your core engaged, lift the hips to Dolphin Plank. Hold the plank for 3-5 full breaths. Slowly and with control, lower back to Sphinx Pose. Complete a total of five repetitions.

Cautions: avoid this pose if you are suffering from a recent or chronic back, arm or shoulder injury, or are in the 2nd or 3rd trimester of pregnancy.

Benefits: strengthens the spine, core and glutes; stretches the front torso and shoulders; stimulates abdominal organs; helps to relieve stress.

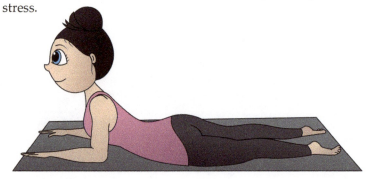

Cobra Pose (*Bhujangasana*)

Lie face down on your mat with your legs extended out behind you. Your feet should be a few inches apart, the tops of your feet down on the mat and your toes should be pointing straight back (not in towards each other). Bring your palms to the mat just below your shoulders, elbows in close to your sides. While pressing down through your feet, legs and pelvis, begin to press through your hands, lifting your shoulders and chest up off the mat into a backbend. Straighten your arms only as much as you can while keeping your pelvis down on the mat, being careful not to bend too sharply in the lower back. Stay long through the neck and open through the chest, making sure to keep your shoulders down and away from the ears. Hold for 3-5 breaths and release.

Variation/Modification: for more ease through the lower back, try walking your hands out further away from you, placing a folded-up blanket under your belly, or holding Baby Cobra, by keeping a strong bend in the elbows.

Cautions: in the case of back injuries, stay low, keeping your elbows bent and tucked in at your sides; avoid this pose if you are in your 2nd or 3rd trimester of pregnancy.

Benefits: stretches the chest, abs and shoulders; strengthens the spine; improves spine mobility and digestion; helps to relieve stress, fatigue and symptoms of sciatica.

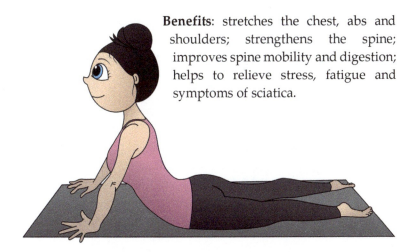

Four Limbed Staff Pose (*Chaturanga Dandasana*)

Begin in Plank Pose. Tighten up through your shoulders, back, core and legs. Shift your weight forward onto your tippy toes. On your exhale, slowly and with control, lower your body by bending your elbows, keeping your arms tucked firmly to the sides of your torso. Stay strong through the body and avoid dipping your belly down or spiking your hips up. Gaze can stay down at your mat or be taken forward ahead of you. Hold for 1-3 breaths. To release, allow yourself to lower gently down onto your mat. Alternatively, you can press back to Downward Facing Dog, or transition to Upward Facing Dog.

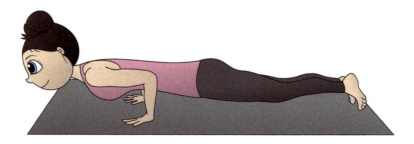

Variation/Modification: this pose is often practised as part of the Sun Salutations sequences. It can be difficult for beginners and experienced yogis alike. To safely modify this pose when transitioning to Upward Facing Dog or Cobra, begin from a Plank position, try Eight Limb Pose (*Ashtanga Namaskara*), shown below. Shift forward on your toes, gently lower your knees down, then bend your elbows keeping them close to your sides as you bring your chin down to the mat, gazing forward. From here you can transition to a backbend. If you are holding the pose, shift your weight forward in Plank, gently lower your knees to the mat, then lower your chest to a few inches above the mat, arms tucked to your sides, gaze forward (like the lower part of a modified push-

Chaturanga continued...

up). To release, return to Plank Pose, transition to Downward Facing Dog, or press back to Child's Pose.

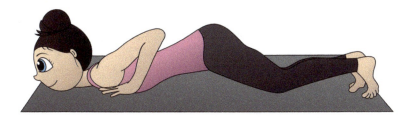

Cautions: avoid this pose if you are suffering from a wrist injury/condition, a shoulder injury, or are in the 2nd or 3rd trimester of pregnancy; if you have a neck injury, keep your gaze down at the mat and avoid gazing forward.

Benefits: strengthens the wrists, arms, shoulders, back and abdomen.

Upward Facing Dog Pose (*Urdhva Mukha Svanasana*)

Begin lying face-down on your mat, feet hip width apart. Make sure your toes are pointing straight back and not in towards each other. Place your hands down at your sides at waist level, just above the navel. Spread your fingers wide, pressing your fingertips into the mat. On an inhale, press through your hands and lift your chest up off the mat, followed by your belly, hips and thighs, pressing down through the tops of your feet. There should be a space between your thighs and the mat. Stay strong through your arms, shoulders and legs. Keep your shoulders low, to allow length through the cervical spine. Squeeze your core, lifting your navel towards your spine and sending your tailbone down towards your pelvis. Gaze forward or slightly up. Be careful not to compress the neck. Hold for 3-5 breaths. To release, lower back down to the mat or transition to Downward Facing Dog. Other ways to enter this pose include lowering the hips from Plank Pose, or lifting through the front body from Four-Limbed Staff Pose (such as in a Sun Salutation sequence).

Variation/Modification: to assist in raising your thighs off the mat, place a rolled-up blanket just below your hips at the tops of your thighs. Alternatively you can practise Cobra Pose in place of Upward Facing Dog.

Cautions: avoid this pose if you are suffering from a wrist or back injury, if you are experiencing headaches or dizziness, or if you are in the 2nd or 3rd trimesters of pregnancy; for neck injuries, avoid gazing up.

Benefits: strengthens the wrists, arms, spine and glutes; stretches the front torso and shoulders; stimulates abdominal organs; helps to improve posture and relieve sciatica.

Child's Pose (*Balasana*)

Kneel on your mat with your big toes together and your knees apart, almost as wide as your mat. Send your sit bones back over your heels as you bend your torso forward from the hips between your thighs. Keep reaching your tailbone back as you extend through your neck, pulling your head away from your shoulders. Your arms may come to rest at your sides, palms facing up. Alternatively you can extend your arms out ahead of you, stretching through the shoulders, chest and upper back. Hold for 30 seconds or longer.

Variation/Modification: if you have tight hips, bring your knees together. If your wrists are sore from your practice, you can use this time to rotate and stretch them. If you're feeling pressure in your knees, try Extended Puppy Pose by keeping your knees bent to a 90° angle, as in Table Pose, lowering your heart to the mat as you outstretch your arms ahead of you.

Cautions: avoid this pose if you have a knee injury or modify to Extended Puppy Pose; in 2nd & 3rd trimesters of pregnancy, keep your knees spread wide to relieve pressure on the abdomen.

Benefits: stretches the hips, thighs and ankles, softly stretches the back; relaxes the muscles in the front of the body; has a calming effect on the body; stimulates digestion.

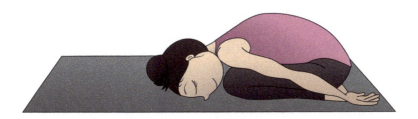

Staff Pose (*Dandasana*)

Sit on your mat with your legs together, outstretched in front of you. Keep your feet flexed as you reach out from your heels. Adjust your pelvis so that your sit bones connect comfortably to the floor without your torso leaning forward or back. Engage a slight inner rotation through your thighs as you press them down towards your mat. Tuck your navel as you lift through the front torso. Ground through the back torso, keep your shoulders down and back, and your tailbone reaching to the floor. Stay long in the neck, keeping your chin parallel to the mat. Position your hands down on the mat at the sides of your thighs or hips. Hold for 3-10 breaths.

Variation/Modification: if you are uncomfortable in Staff Pose due to tightness through the back of your legs, try sitting on a blanket or cushion to raise the hips.

Cautions: if you have a wrist injury, avoid pressing your hands into the mat, lay them gently on your lap instead; avoid this pose if you have a lower back injury.

Benefits: strengthens the back; stretches the shoulders and chest; improves posture and concentration; helps to relieve stress.

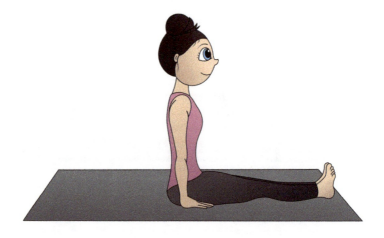

Seated Forward Fold (*Paschimottanasana*)

Sitting in Staff Pose (legs extended out ahead of you, feet together), inhale your arms up and overhead, lengthening through your spine. On your exhale, begin to fold forward from the hips. Keep your back straight and bring your belly to the tops of your thighs, followed by your chest and then your chin and nose. Hold onto your shins, toes or ankles, bending the knees as much as you need to (until your flexibility improves). On each inhale, lengthen through the front torso and on the exhale, bend a little deeper. Hold for 3-5 breaths.

Variation/Modification: to relieve stress and tightness in the lower back/hamstrings, place a blanket or cushion beneath your tush.

Cautions: if you have back pain or a mild back injury, make sure to keep your back as straight as possible and avoid folding forward too low; for shoulder injuries, keep your arms down, sitting up as tall as you can before folding over; avoid this pose if you are experiencing diarrhea or have a severe back injury.

Benefits: stretches the back, shoulders, pelvis and hamstrings; relieves cramps and stress; improves digestion; reduces anxiety and fatigue; stimulates the liver, kidneys, adrenal glands, ovaries and uterus.

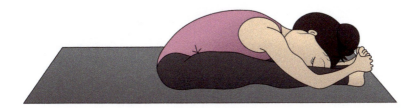

Bridge Pose (*Setu Bandha Sarvangasana*)

Lie flat on your back with your knees bent, arms at your sides. Line your feet up beneath your knees, hip width apart. On an inhale, engage your core and legs and raise your pelvis up until your thighs are about parallel to the mat and also to each other. Focus on keeping your hips elevated with your leg muscles more so than your glutes. Raise your chin slightly and gaze towards the ceiling. You can keep your arms at your sides or shift your upper body from side to side to bring your shoulder blades closer together, clasping your hands beneath your tush. Hold for 3-5 breaths, then release on an exhale.

Variation/Modification: place a block between your thighs as you hold this pose to help you connect to your leg muscles and to encourage proper alignment in the legs and feet.

Cautions: avoid this pose if you have a neck or shoulder injury.

Benefits: strengthens the legs and glutes; stretches the chest, neck and back; stimulates the abdominal organs; helps to reduce stress, back pain and headaches.

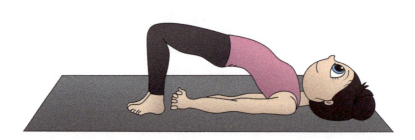

Wind Relieving Pose (*Pavanamuktasana*)

Lie on your back with your legs extended out straight (you can also get there from a bent knee position, such as in Bridge Pose). On an exhale, draw both knees towards your chest placing your hands on your knees/shins, being careful not to curl the tailbone up. Get heavy through your sacrum (a bone in the lowest part of your back just above the tailbone) and shoulders allowing them to sink into the mat. Maintain a neutral spine as much as possible. Tuck your chin down slightly to lengthen the neck. You can hold here for 3-10 steady breaths, or proceed to Half Wind Relieving Pose on either side: from Wind Relieving Pose, hold on to your right knee as you extend your left leg out long onto the mat, nodding your chin down to lengthen the neck as your head lifts up off the mat. Hold this position for 3-5 breaths, then repeat on the other side.

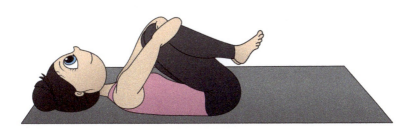

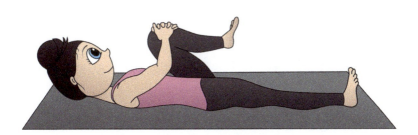

Wind Relieving Pose continued...

Variation/Modification: if you have difficulty reaching your knees without lifting your head off the mat, try placing a blanket under your head (but not your neck); if you have a neck injury, avoid nodding the chin down and keep your head down on the mat.

Cautions: avoid this pose if you have a hernia, have had a recent abdominal procedure, have had a recent back injury or have sciatica; for knee issues, place your hands under your knees on the backs of your thighs to hold this pose or avoid this pose altogether, keeping your feet on the mat, arms at your sides.

Benefits: stretches the back; reduces stress, anxiety, bloating and flatulence; improves concentration, digestion and gas emissions.

Corpse Pose (*Savasana*)

Lie on your mat, flat on your back with your arms resting at your sides and your legs outstretched. That's it. Just kidding! Sometimes used at the beginning of a class, Savasana is most often done at the end of your practice. This pose is all about relaxation, which can be surprisingly difficult. You want your body to be resting in a neutral position without any tension. Begin with your pelvis, making sure it's not tilted forward. Reach down through your tailbone to adjust it. Then allow your legs to turn out comfortably, feet resting as they may, hip width apart or wider. Widen your shoulder blades and turn your arms, palms facing up. Don't be afraid to take up space, however, try to stay on your mat. If your limbs come off your mat, be mindful of your neighbour. Close your eyes. Next, mentally scan your body from your toes to the top of your head searching for any tension that needs to be released. Adjust your body as necessary. Be extra mindful of your neck, throat, jaw and brow as these areas tend to be very tense. Feel yourself getting heavy as you allow every part of your body to sink into the mat. Breathe deeply and evenly. Tune out external distractions and focus your mind on a single thought, mantra or your breath. Stay in this pose for 3-10 minutes. To release, wake up the body slowly by wiggling your toes, making fists with your hands and fluttering the eyes open. Take your time coming to a seated position before standing.

Variation/Modification: if you are uncomfortable lying flat on your back because of a neck or back pain or any other reason, you can place a cushion or blanket beneath your head and/or a pillow or rolled-up blanket under your knees to allow for complete relaxation.

Cautions: avoid lying flat on your back if you're in your 2nd or 3rd trimester of pregnancy. Instead, turn onto your left side and place a cushion under your head for support, keeping your hips stacked, knees slightly bent.

Savasana continued...

Benefits: increases concentration, focus, energy levels and self-awareness; relieves stress, anxiety and symptoms of depression; reduces headaches; aids in muscle recuperation; leaves the practitioner feeling reinvigorated.

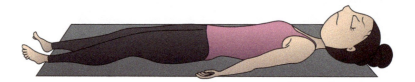

Sun Salutations (*Surya Namaskar*)

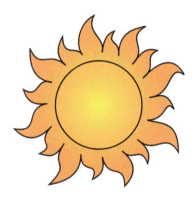

Surya = Sun
Namaskar = The act of bringing your palms together in prayer and bowing to show respect.

The sun is our main source of life and light. It holds a strong place in ancient and modern day scriptures and philosophies and is symbolic in many cultures. We love the sun. The sun is great! And so to honour the sun, we do Sun Salutations.

Sun Salutations are best practised in the morning at sunrise. I'm not the boss of you though, so you can practise them anytime you want. However, Sun Salutation sequences are meant to wake you up and get you energized. They are therefore performed at the beginning of a class.

Over the years (we're talking well over 2,000 years) the sequence of postures that make up the Sun Salutations has varied. The flow may differ from school to school, studio to studio. The Classical Sun Salutation which most seem to agree upon is:

Classical Sun Salutation

Mountain Pose

Upward Salute

Standing Forward Fold

Half Standing Forward Fold

Standing Forward Fold

Low Lunge, right foot back, arms up

Plank Pose

Four-Limbed Staff Pose

Upward-Facing Dog Pose

Downward-Facing Dog Pose

Step right foot through between hands

Low Lunge, right leg forward, arms up

Transition – feet to hands

Half Standing Forward Fold

Standing Forward Fold

Upward Salute

Mountain Pose

Classical Sun Salutation
(*Surya Namaskar*)

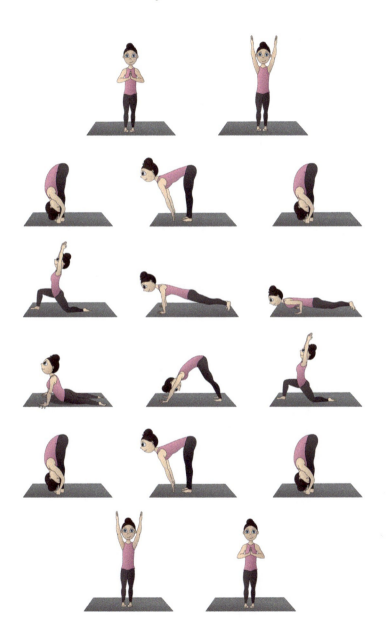

There are two variations of the Classical Sun Salutation that are most prevalent today:

Sun Salutation Variation A:

Mountain Pose

Upward Salute

Standing Forward Fold

Standing Half Forward Fold

Standing Forward Fold

Plank Pose

Four-Limbed Staff

Upward-Facing Dog Pose

Downward-Facing Dog Pose

Transition – feet to hands

Standing Half Forward Fold

Standing Forward Fold

Upward Salute

Mountain Pose

Sun Salutation Variation B:

Mountain Pose
Chair Pose
Standing Forward Fold
Half Standing Forward Fold
Standing Forward Fold
Plank Pose
Four-Limbed Staff
Upward-Facing Dog
Downward-Facing Dog
Right foot forward to Warrior I
Plank Pose
Four-Limbed Staff
Upward-Facing Dog
Downward-Facing Dog
Left foot forward to Warrior I
Plank Pose
Four-Limbed Staff
Upward-Facing Dog
Downward-Facing Dog
Transition – feet to hands
Half Standing Forward Fold
Standing Forward Fold
Chair Pose
Mountain Pose

Sun Salutation variations may differ slightly depending on who is teaching them, but you get the gist of it. And trust me, take enough vinyasa-style classes and you'll be doing Sun Salutations in your sleep! At the start of a class you may do anywhere from 3-5 in a row to start, working your way up to even more.

As you move through the sequences, you are to flow with your breath. That is to say you are to move with each breath. For example, from Mountain Pose, inhale your arms up to Upward Salute, then exhale into Standing Forward Bend. Inhale to Standing Half Forward Bend, exhale, return to Standing Forward Bend, and so on. It is important to note that as you move, your body heats up and your heart rate increases which causes you to breathe faster. Since you're moving with your breath, this may result in you performing the Sun Salutations more and more quickly. Be aware of this. Focus on keeping a slow and steady breath.

Performing Sun Salutations helps to quickly connect you to your body and breath. They are great to get you into "the zone". Like a warm-up. Actually, I like to think of Sun Salutations as the burpees of the yoga world. Think about it, a full body warm-up that serves as a workout at the same time. The movement lines sort of resemble each other...is it just me? OK.

Fun fact: the number of rounds traditionally practised is 108 Sun Salutations. What!?!? That's right. Though in today's world this number may not be something we do every day or even every week. Who's got the time? You will see special classes pop up around the change of seasons throughout the year in which you will be guided through the 108 as a class. It is usually Sun Salutation A that is repeated 108 times.. If this is something you plan to participate in, try to avoid an upper body workout before and after the scheduled Sun Salutations. Trust me, you need your upper body strength to get through them, and you are definitely going to be feeling it after! Don't let lack of experience discourage you from trying one of these classes out. You may learn a lot about yourself and about yoga. If you're intimidated by the volume of asana to be done, you can always take a break during the class by holding Mountain Pose or Child's Pose to rest, then jumping back in when you're ready. You may notice others in the class doing the same!

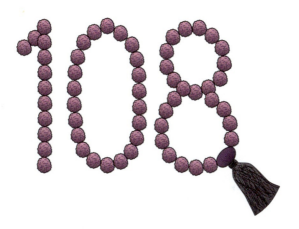

Why 108? The number 108 pops up everywhere in yoga. I mean everywhere. It's a little freaky. So much so that in yoga, 108 is considered a sacred number. To list just a few examples:

- The diameter of the sun is 108 times that of the Earth;
- The distance between the Earth and the sun is 108 times the diameter of the sun;
- According to Ayurvedic teachings, there are 108 marma points (pressure points) in the body;
- The human body contains 108 nadis (energy channels);
- Malas (a set of prayer beads to count mantras) are traditionally made up of 108 beads.
- The volume of asanas repeated challenges the yogi mentally and physically allowing them to discover things about themselves and rid themselves of unwanted feelings and emotions giving new meaning to their practice. It is believed to have a cleansing effect on the body, mind and soul.

When to practise 108? Anytime, anywhere. Today it is most commonly done at the change of the season: Spring Equinox, Summer Solstice, Autumnal Equinox and Winter Solstice. As we reflect upon the season past, we welcome the change and growth with the new season to come.

Now, you've heard of Sun Salutations, but what about the moon? Of course there are Moon Salutation sequences (*Chandra Namaskar*, *Chandra* = Moon). Where the Sun Salutations fire you up, Moon Salutations are meant to calm you down. They are best practised near the end of a class, before meditation, before bedtime or anytime that you need to cool off.

Resembling a lunar cycle in its progression, a typical Moon Salutation goes something like this (though as with Sun Salutations, there are multiple variations):

Moon Salutation
(Facing the long edge of the mat)

Mountain Pose
Raise your arms overhead
Standing Side Bend, right side
Five Pointed Star Pose
Goddess Pose
Triangle Pose on the right side
Rotate to Pyramid Pose, right leg forward
Drop the left knee
Lift the arms to Low Lunge
Lower the hands down to the mat
Transition - Rotate to face the long edge of the mat
Deep Side Squat (right knee bent)
Garland Pose

Reverse the sequence coming back up on the left side and ending in Mountain Pose.

Moon Salutation
(*Chandra Namaskar*)

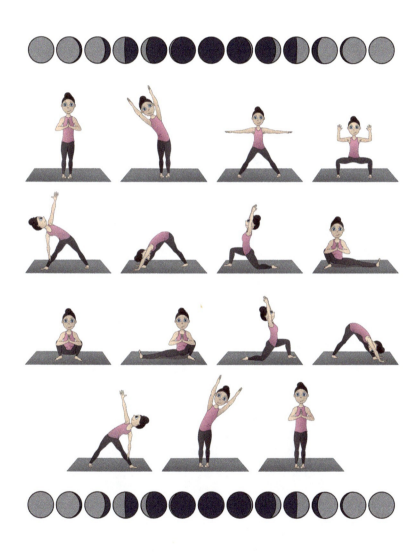

This sequence can be repeated as many times as you feel is right to get to where you want to be. Yoga is about getting to know yourself and your body. So it's important that during your practice you stay tuned in. Pay attention to how your movements are making you feel physically, mentally and emotionally. Since yoga is also about finding your bliss, do what feels right for you.

With any vinyasa (flow) you should match your breath to your movements. In yoga we inhale as we open up through the torso and exhale as we close up (bends and twists). In a flowy, more fast paced sequence, it can be difficult to link up our breath to these types of poses, so if you're not sure, just do what feels right. Alternating an inhale and an exhale with each movement is the rule of thumb, but if you're not there yet or it feels unnatural to you, just focus on maintaining a strong, steady breath.

How quickly you move through each sequence depends on a few factors.

Your breath: if you are practising at your own pace, each movement of the sequence should correspond to the length of your natural breath. This may be slower to start and then slightly pick up as you get moving.

Your goals: if you are looking for a heart pumping cardio session, move through your sequence more quickly. If you want to tone and strengthen, slow it down. If you are looking for a calming, soothing experience, move at a gentle pace.

Your surroundings: some classes encourage you to move at your own pace. But when you have a certain number of sequences to get through in one class, you will be encouraged to keep up with those around you. Moving with a class can be fun and challenging, forcing you to change your natural pace. It almost feels like a dance!

Your time: these types of sequences are great for squeezing in some yoga asana when you are short on time while still feeling like you got a good practice in. Pop out 10 Sun Salutations when you wake up and you'll still be left with plenty of time to put your face on.

Your appetite: just ate a bit meal? You're not going to get through a lot of rounds of any sequence, and certainly not quickly. Sun Salutations, Moon Salutations as with most yoga classes and posture sequences are best practised after a light meal or on an empty (or close to) stomach.

EIGHT

Pranaya-Wha?

Pranayama is one of The Eight Limbs of Yoga as described by Patanjali. It is an essential component of your yoga practice, enabling you to further control your physical body, your mental faculties and your emotional well-being. Your breath is your life's force and thus should be afforded as much importance as every other part of your practice. Ignore it, and your physical performance, focus and concentration will begin to suffer while your emotions get the better of you.

The practice of yoga leads to a healthy body inside and out. Consider incorporating breathing techniques into your regular self-care routine and you will soon see improvements to your everyday life.

The benefits of pranayama include increased lung capacity, the ability to hold your breath for longer periods of time and improved function of the respiratory system. You'll experience increased oxygen intake which leads to increases in energy, focus, concentration, improved cognitive and nerve function, and reduced buildup of lactic acid throughout the body. Pranayama boosts immunity, decreases stress and anxiety and relieves insomnia.

It is important to begin your pranayama practice slowly. Many techniques involve interrupted breathing which may lead to stress if approached too vigorously. If you experience dizziness, nausea, shortness of breath, a headache or discomfort of any kind, you should reduce your efforts and modify where you can. If these symptoms persist, stop practising the techniques that are causing them until you've developed a higher tolerance to the more basic breathing patterns.

There are many types of pranayama. From natural breathing to interrupted breathing, there are techniques for all types of practice. Some are used for meditation, while others are great for a fast-paced vinyasa flow. Simply turning your attention to your breath is a breathing technique. You know when you're upset about something and someone else annoyingly tells you to take some deep breaths? Yeah, there's something to that.

Here are some techniques that you might find most useful.

Note: avoid practising the intermediate and advanced level techniques until you are comfortable enough at the beginner level to proceed.

Dirgha Pranayama
a.k.a.: Complete Breath, Three Part Breath
Level: beginner/all levels

To practise: Sit comfortably with your abdomen relaxed. Inhale deeply through both nostrils as you feel your belly expand all the way around. Continue to inhale, feeling the air fill your lungs as your chest, then collar bones begin to rise. Pause. Take in just a touch more air. On the exhale, reverse the order: first feel your collar bones lower, then your chest, and finally your abdomen compressing as you release every last bit of air. Practise this technique during your asana practice when you're holding a seated posture, at the start of a relaxing reclined posture, before meditation, before you go to sleep at night or any time during the day when you may feel anxious, stressed or angry.

Ujjayi Pranayama
a.k.a.: Ujjayi Breath, Victorious Breath, Conqueror Breath, Ocean Breath
Level: beginner/all levels

To practise: Ujjayi breath is most often performed throughout your asana practice. The depth of this technique will strengthen your practice as it reduces stress and increases energy, focus and concentration. The idea here is to lightly constrict the opening at the top of your throat as you draw out long, strong inhales and exhales. When you first begin, inhale through both nostrils, and exhale through your mouth slightly open. With practice, you will feel comfortable completing the entire breath with your mouth closed. This breath should not feel forced, but rather somewhat relaxed. If you're feeling faint and not getting enough air, you're constricting the throat too much, try easing up. As you constrict the throat, you will feel the base of your tongue widen and lower. The resulting sound should be similar to ocean waves. Start with an inhale of three seconds, and work on being able to increase that over time. Your exhale should last as long as your inhale, or longer, but never shorter. Since this breath is used as you're moving around, you may draw shorter and longer breaths all throughout the same sequence; quicker breaths during a fast paced flow, then slowing the breath down as you hold a pose for a bit longer.

Nadi Shodhana
a.k.a.: Anulom Vilom, Alternate Nostril Breathing
Level: beginner/all levels

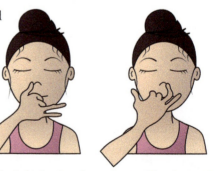

To practise: Sit up tall and get long through the neck, keeping your chin parallel to the floor, or slightly nodded down. Lay your left hand comfortably on your left knee or in your lap. At the end of an exhale, close your right nostril with your right thumb. Inhale slowly and steadily through the left nostril. At the top of the inhale, pause, close the left nostril with your right ring finger, and exhale slowly through the right nostril. At the end of the exhale, inhale through the right nostril. At the top of the inhale, pause, close the right nostril with your thumb. Exhale, then inhale through the left nostril. Continue, alternating sides during the pause at the top of each inhale until you've completed five full breaths through each nostril. This technique is believed to cleanse the energy channels in the body (nadis) to ease the flow of breath throughout our practice.

Surya/Chandra Bhedana Pranayama
a.k.a.: Single Nostril Breath, Sun Piercing Breath (Surya Bhedana), Moon Piercing Breath (Chandra Bhedana)
Level: beginner/all levels

To practise: The right side of your body is represented by the sun (Surya). Energetically, it is the masculine side of the body, bringing energy and heat. The left side of your body is represented by the moon (Chandra). It is the feminine side of the body, creative, calming and cool. Focusing the flow of air through just one nostril allows us to draw energy from that side of the body. If you feel low on energy and need a little fire, practise Surya Bhedana. If you're feeling anxious or need to cool down, practise Chandra Bhedana. To practise Surya Bhedana, sit up tall and get long through the neck, keeping your chin parallel to the floor, or slightly nodded down. Lay your left hand comfortably on your left knee or in your lap. At the end of an exhale, close your left nostril with your right ring finger and inhale deeply and with control through your right nostril. Pause. Close your right nostril with your right thumb and exhale through your left nostril. Repeat this pattern, inhaling only through the right side for 5-10 rounds. Pause at the top of each inhale. The duration of the pause may lengthen with practice. Once you've gotten used to holding it for one second, increase the pause slowly over time for as long as you feel comfortable holding it, without having to burst out, and exhale afterwards. To practise Chandra Bhedana, reverse the nostril alternating of the Surya Bhedana, so that you are inhaling only through the left nostril, and exhaling through the right.

Kumbhaka Pranayama
a.k.a.: Breath Retention
Level: intermediate to advanced

To practise: This technique may be practised at the end of an inhale (Antara Kumbhaka) for intermediate-level practitioners or at the end of an exhale (Bahya Kumbhaka) for more advanced yogis. Either way, the part of the breath at the end of which the breath is held should be exaggerated. If holding at the end of an inhale, inhale a little deeper than you normally would for an ordinary breath. If holding at the end of an exhale, exhale more than you normally would, emptying the lungs as much as you can. To start, from a seated position, engage Mula Bandha (root lock) and Jalandhara Bandha (chin lock) - see Chapter 9. Antara Kumbhaka: take a deep inhale and then hold your breath for 3-10 seconds. Exhale with control and then return to your regular breath or to ujjayi breathing for three full breaths. Repeat for up to five minutes. Bahya Kumbhaka: following a long exhale, hold your breath for 3-10 seconds. Inhale slowly and then return to your regular breath or to ujjayi breathing for three full breaths. Repeat for up to five minutes. The length of retention depends on your level or practice. When you release the hold, you should not burst an exhale or gasp an inhale. If this is the case, hold your breath for a shorter amount of time. Be extra cautious with breath retention. Stop immediately if you feel dizzy or faint. Kumbhaka Pranayama helps to decrease stress, improve energy levels, mental focus and respiratory health.

Kapalabhati Pranayama
a.k.a.: Breath of Fire, Cleansing Breath, Skull Shining Breath
Level: intermediate/advanced

To practise: The focus of this technique is on the exhale. Sit in an upright position on your mat or a chair. Place your hands on your knees, or folded over your lower belly. Inhale naturally and deeply through the nostrils. Contract your abdomen, pulling your navel towards your spine, and exhale in a short, quick burst.

Repeat for one minute. Aim for 40-50 breath cycles per minute to start, working your way up to 100 cycles per minute in five cycle increments. Kapalabhati can help to clear the bronchial passages, the lungs and the sinuses, helping to relieve and prevent related illnesses and allergies.

Bhastrika Pranayama
a.k.a.: Bellows Breath
Level: intermediate/advanced

To practise: The focus of this technique is to breathe forcefully on the inhale and the exhale. Sit comfortably in an upright position, folding your hands over your belly. Take a few natural breaths and focus on the feeling of your abdomen expanding and contracting. Begin by exhaling powerfully through both nostrils as you contract your abdomen towards your spine. Immediately inhale through the nostrils, feeling your belly press against your hands with force. Start with breaths that are about 2-3 seconds per inhale and exhale, making them even in duration. Over time, reduce the length of each inhale and exhale to one second each. Repeat for 5-10 rounds, increasing the number of rounds over time until you can comfortably breathe this way for one full minute. Avoid this practice if you are pregnant, suffer from hypertension, epilepsy, anxiety or panic disorder. Stop if you begin to feel dizzy or nauseous. This technique is best practised in the morning, before a strenuous activity, or any time that you need to feel energized and invigorated.

Sitali Pranayama
a.k.a.: Cooling Breath, Sheetali Pranayama
Level: beginner/all levels/limited to those who can curl their tongues

To practise: Sit comfortably in proper alignment, staying long through the neck. Curl your tongue and stick it out just past your lips. Inhale slowly, feeling your belly expand and focusing on the coolness of the air as it passes over your tongue. Close your mouth and exhale through your nostrils. Continue this pattern for 1-2 minutes. Return to natural breathing for 2-3 minutes. Repeat the Cooling Breath one more time. With practice, work your way up to five minutes of continuous Sitali Pranayama. The breath drawn over a wet tongue brings moisture into your system. This technique is said to stave off hunger and temporarily quench thirst. It is physically cooling and beneficial on hot days, when experiencing fever or hot flashes. It helps to calm anger and prevent foul breath.

Sitkari Pranayama
a.k.a.: Hissing Breath
Level: beginner/all levels

To practise: Sit comfortably in proper alignment, staying long through the neck. Touch your tongue to the back of your front teeth, keeping your jaw closed. Gently separate your lips and inhale slowly through clenched teeth. You should hear a light hissing sound. Close your lips and exhale through your nose. Continue this pattern for 1-2 minutes. Return to your natural breath for 2-3 minutes. Repeat the Hissing Breath one more time. With practice, work your way up to five minutes of continuous Sitkari Pranayama. This technique is a great alternative to the Sitali Pranayama if you are unable to curl your tongue. It has a cooling effect on the body, helps to prevent ailments of the mouth and throat and helps to reduce high blood pressure.

Bhramari Pranayama
a.k.a.: Bee Breath
Level: beginner/all levels

To practise: In a calm quiet place, sit comfortably upright with a straight back. Tuck your chin down towards your chest and get long in the back of the neck. Place your index fingers on the tragus of each ear (the cartilage between the ear and cheek that partly covers the ear canal). Alternatively, you can place your thumbs over your tragi and cover your eyes/brow with your fingers. Keep your mouth closed, teeth together or slightly apart with your tongue up against the back of your top front teeth. Inhale through the nose, then as you exhale, make a humming sound from the back of the throat. Repeat this pattern for 1-2 minutes. Return to your natural breath for 2-3 minutes. Repeat the Bee Breath one more time. With practice, work your way up to five minutes of continuous Bhramari Pranayama. Avoid this technique if you are pregnant, suffering from epilepsy or an ear infection. Bee Breath is very effective in quickly calming the mind and nerves, relieving tension, reducing stress, anxiety and anger and strengthening vocal abilities.

Having control over your breath by practising these techniques regularly and with attention throughout your yoga practice can benefit you immensely in your everyday life. Without even realizing it, you'll begin to use breath to calm yourself in stressful situations every day. You may even find yourself getting to sleep quicker at night. Other forms of exercise may become easier as you apply this practice to running, cycling, weight lifting, etc. And for the expectant mother, breath control will serve you well through labour.

Be mindful of your breath. When we're not, we may find ourselves taking shallow, irregular breaths that do not serve us. Take the time throughout your day to focus on your breath and it will become second nature. We do not need to be sitting on our yoga mats to practise breathing techniques. Sitting at your desk at work after your boss has pissed you off for the third time that day is just as good a time as any!

NINE

Bandhas

Practising breathing techniques allows us to expand our vital life force energy throughout our bodies. Bandhas (body locks), practised together with pranayama, direct that life force energy to specific areas of the body.

There are four types of bandhas, each one linked to a channel within the body to which energy may be directed. Bandhas help to add power, concentration, stability and focus to your practice. To practise a bandha means to contract a specific set of muscles (an internal lock).

Bandhas may be practised on their own, with breathing techniques, or with poses and are incorporated throughout the practice of asana and pranayama in preparation for meditation.

The four bandhas are:

Mula Bandha: (Root Lock) This bandha involves the contraction and lifting of the perineum and the surrounding muscles that make up the pelvic floor. As we contract this set of muscles, we should imagine bringing them all in towards a centre point, while lifting them up. Think about having to hold in your pee, or doing kegels. It's kind of like that but it involves a slightly broader area. Mula Bandha brings energy to your root and sends it upwards, awakening the kundalini power (or Shakti energy) at the base of your spine. This bandha stimulates the pelvic muscles and nerves, the genital organs and excretory system. It is especially beneficial to the expectant mother to learn how to control the muscles of the pelvic floor so that she may relax them when the time comes to release her human creation into the world. It assists well in back bends and is often paired with Uddiyana Bandha in balance poses.

It should be avoided in forward bends as in these poses we want to widen through the seat and therefore must relax the pelvic floor.

<u>To practise</u>: engage your root lock at the end of an inhale and hold the lock for three full breaths, releasing on an exhale. Take five full breaths, then repeat. With time, increase the duration of the hold.

Uddiyana Bandha: (Abdominal Lock) This powerful bandha continues to bring that energy up from your root and towards your heart. Uddiyana Bandha involves contracting the abdominal muscles in and up. This is not to be confused with "engaging your core" as we do in many forms of exercise since the abdominal lock focuses strictly on the front of the torso. It is super fun to say and has many benefits that make it worth practising. This bandha tones the abdominal muscles, stretches the diaphragm, stimulates the abdominal organs, improves digestion, promotes improved function of the adrenal glands, relieves constipation, stress and tension, and boosts metabolism. Avoid this lock if you are pregnant, menstruating, or are suffering from ulcers, a hernia or high blood pressure. It is best practised on an empty stomach. Mula Bandha and Uddiyana Bandha are often practised together as it can be difficult to separate the two, although this is a great skill to acquire. When practised together, you will feel as though your breath is coming from down low as you notice your ribcage expand with each breath. Avoid the abdominal lock in backbends as you want to relax this set of muscles so that they can fully expand and lend to the pose. Uddiyana Bandha pairs well with balance poses, one-legged balance poses and arm balances.

<u>To practise</u>: lie flat on your back, legs outstretched, arms at your sides. As you exhale, contract your abdominal muscles in and up as much as you can. At the very end of your exhale, hold your breath. You should feel that there is a hollow in your gut. Hold for 3-5 seconds, then release on an inhale. Work your way up to longer holds over time.

Note: Some asanas will require you to engage your core. While your instructor may refer to this as the abdominal lock, or Uddiyana Bandha, keep in mind that although the two seem to be interchangeable in yoga practice, there is a difference. Your core comprises the muscles from the bottom of your glutes, all the way up to your ribcage. It includes your abdominals, the muscles of your mid and lower back and all those that wrap around your torso. In Uddiyana Bandha, only the abdominals are involved in the lock and therefore your spine may remain unstable, possibly adding strain to an otherwise safe pose. For example, when holding Plank Pose, you want to fully engage your core, being sure to remain strong through the lower back. If you don't, your belly may dip no matter how strongly you're pulling in your navel, sending you into a backbend. The abdominal lock possesses many benefits and is a great start to engaging your core. But if you are looking for something to give you more stability, engage your core instead. To do this, imagine a girdle around your waist squeezing you in. Tighten up all of the muscles that you can connect to (below your sternum and above your pubis) towards the centre of your body. Keep these muscles contracted as you breathe during poses such as Plank Pose, Four-Limbed Staff Pose, Warrior II, and others. So when you're in class, and your instructor says Uddiyana Bandha, and you feel like you need more: Engage. Your. Core. Please.

Jalandhara Bandha: (Chin Lock) Sometimes called throat lock, this bandha involves nodding your chin down towards your chest. It controls the energy flow throughout the neck. Contract your throat muscles as you pull your chin back and down towards your collar bones. You may feel like you have a double chin. This bandha improves thyroid and parathyroid function, calms the autonomic nervous system, helps to regulate the vascular system, respiratory system and the metabolism, and helps to relieve stress and lower blood pressure. It is most often practised before meditation. Avoid this lock if you have a neck injury. A modified chin lock can be used in place where the chin nods down slightly as you lengthen through the back of the neck. This is beneficial in poses such as Wind Relieving Pose, Half Wind Relieving Pose and Child's Pose.

To practise: sit in Easy Pose with your hands on your knees, palms facing up with your indexes and thumbs touching tips (Gyan Mudra - Chapter 10). Alternatively, you can rest your hands palms down on your knees, or fold your hands in your lap. Sit up tall, inhale and engage your chin lock. At the top of an inhale, hold your breath. Hold for 3-5 seconds, then release as you exhale and lift your chin. Work your way up to longer holds over time.

Maha Bandha: (Triple Lock) It is important to be well practised in the other three bandhas before engaging the Maha Bandha. Also called the Supreme Bandha, Maha Bandha is the combination of the three other bandhas performed at once starting with the chin lock, then the abdominal lock and finally the root lock. The benefits gained from this practice are all of those reaped by the others together. It provides a cleansing and awakening experience.

To practise: find a comfortable seated position and press your hands down on your knees. The locks begin at the very end of an exhale, as your breath is held. If needed, take in a bit of air for the chin lock. Hold for as long as you comfortably can. When releasing the Maha Bandha, inhale as you first let go of the root lock, then the abdominal lock and finally, the chin lock. Work your way up to longer holds over time.

MAHA BANDHA

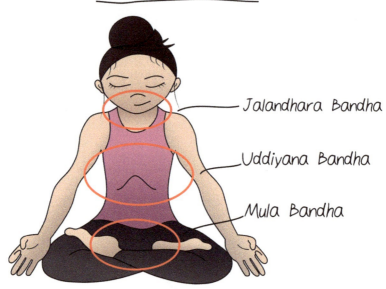

You may or may not be instructed to activate a bandha during your practice. Knowing them, however, can benefit you either way. Certain locks in certain poses may elevate that pose for you and take it to a whole other level. This is something we may not experience if our instructor does not encourage it. Other times, when your instructor does tell you to activate a certain bandha, it may not feel natural to you in that position. In those cases, do what feels right and relax the concentrated area. No one will know the difference and I won't tell. Remember, yoga is a personal practice so you should always do what you feel is best for you.

TEN

Mantras, Mudras & Meditation

Mantras

A mantra is the yogi's catchphrase. But don't have a cow, man! It's not something you need to share with the world.

Simply put, a mantra is a sound, word or phrase that is repeated to help us concentrate in meditation. It may be chanted aloud as a group or alone, muttered under your breath so that only you may hear it, or repeated silently to yourself.

There exist several mantras passed down from ancient scriptures such as the oh-so-popular "OM". Many of them are quite long and require a bit of memorization, so to get started, it's cool to just stick with "OM".

OM: (Pronounced AUM) The sound the universe made when it popped into existence. "OM" means "Source" or "Supreme". Chanting "OM" gives you good vibrations, increased focus and concentration, a sense of calm and helps to purify the space around you.

Alternatively, a mantra may be a personal phrase or slogan, unique to you.

<u>To practise</u>: think of a mantra at the beginning of your practice and pay attention to how it makes you feel. Continue to remind yourself of it through your pranayama, asana and/or meditation. At the end of your practice, summon your mantra and reexamine

the feeling it gives you. Did your practice give you new perspective or improve your emotional state? Was your mantra an empowering phrase that you previously needed to convince yourself of but now believe with conviction? Did you enter your practice anxious or stressed and now find that you're calm and relaxed? Mantras can not only help you figure this out, they can contribute to your transformation.

My fears do not control me.

I am worth it.

I DO have something to wear.

I don't need to go shopping today.

I am enough.

It's OK if the frame hangs crooked.

I am one sexy bitch.

I am strong.

Mmmmbop

I will give kale another chance.

I choose to be happy.

I can stop after one doughnut.

Mudras

Mudras (meaning = seal) are hand gestures that are performed to release and redirect our internal energy. The reflex points in our hands are activated to stimulate the brain and restore balance to the five elements in the body. The more you practise a mudra, the more of its benefits you will experience. Most are practised during meditation, Gyan Mudra being a go-to, or from a seated position during pranayama. Others, like Anjali Mudra and Kali Mudra are also included throughout our asana practice.

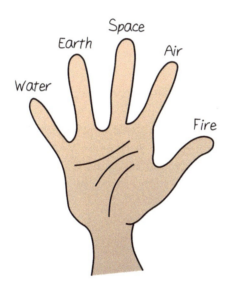

When a mudra includes bringing your hands together, they should be situated near the centre vertical line of the body, unless otherwise directed. When a mudra keeps both hands separate, they would normally be rested on the knees or thighs, palms facing up, with some exceptions, of course.

Choose a mudra that speaks to your needs right now. Really get to know it and stick to it throughout many practices. When holding this mudra, focus on its benefits. Once you've become comfortable with this mudra and its elements or you feel that it has served you fully, become familiar with a new one. There are several mudras and it can be hard to remember them all. This practice can serve as a strategy to expand your knowledge in this area.

Note: Two of the mudras we will see are Surya Mudra and Prithvi Mudra. These two are interchangeable in some schools, and some practise either one or the other. Confusing, right? With so many styles and schools of yoga, it's understandable that we sometimes find contradictions and differences between them. That's OK, practise how you are instructed to, or how you feel is right for you. It's just yoga. Be cool.

Anjali Mudra
a.k.a.: Salutation Seal, The Heart Seal, Prayer Position, Prayer Hands, Namaste Hands
Position: bring the hands together, fingers pointing up, palms and fingertips touching with even pressure through both hands. Rest your thumbs lightly on your sternum, while lifting your sternum towards your thumbs, slightly nod the chin down towards the chest.
Benefits: reduces stress and anxiety; increases concentration and flexibility in the wrists and elbows.

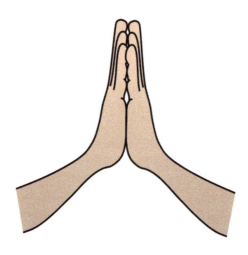

Apana Mudra
a.k.a.: Apan Mudra, Mudra for Digestion, Mudra for Detoxification, Purification Mudra
Position: fold your middle and ring fingers down to meet the tip of the thumb, or rest your thumb lightly over the nails of the two fingers.
Benefits: improves digestion and mental state; helps to cleanse the body of toxins.

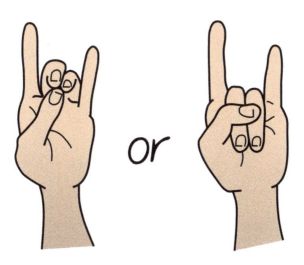

Buddhi Mudra
a.k.a.: Varuna Mudra, Mudra of Water
Position: tips of the thumb and pinky together, other fingers effortlessly extended.
Benefits: improves intuition, mental clarity, digestion, eczema, psoriasis, blood-related conditions, bladder and kidney disorders.

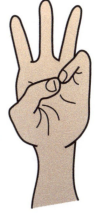

Dhyana Mudra
a.k.a.: Meditation Seal, Mudra for Meditation
Position: palms face-up in your lap stacked right over left, tips of thumbs touching.
Benefits: calms the brain and nerves; increases concentration; creates balance between the two sides of the body.

Gyan Mudra
a.k.a.: Chin Mudra, Consciousness Seal, Mudra of Knowledge
Position: tips of thumb and index fingers together, other fingers may be straight or relaxed.
Benefits: helps to increase concentration, focus and memory retention.

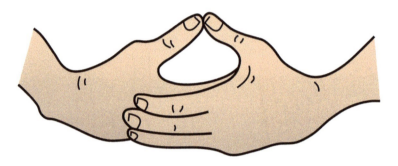

Kali Mudra
a.k.a.: Steeple Hands, Charlie's Angels Mudra
Position: interlace your fingers, keeping your indexes extended and pressed against each other, thumbs crossed.
Benefits: empowering; increases confidence and inner strength; relieves tension; stretches the shoulder and chest and back when arms are extended up.

Padma Mudra
a.k.a.: Lotus Seal, Lotus Mudra
Position: start in Anjali Mudra with your thumbs pointing towards your chest, gently open through the index, middle, then ring fingers, separating them while keeping the thumbs, base of the palms and pinkies together.
Benefits: promotes purity, kindness, compassion, joy and empathy; relaxes and calms the mind.

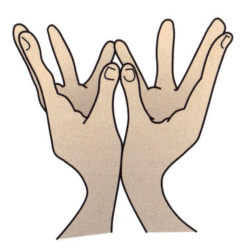

Prana Mudra

a.k.a.: Life Force Seal, Mudra of Life

Position: touch the ring and pinky fingers to the tip of the thumb, other fingers remain extended.

Benefits: increases strength, focus and energy; restores vitality; improves immunity.

Prithvi Mudra

a.k.a.: Mudra of Earth. Some schools view it as being the same as Surya Mudra.

Position: tips of the ring finger and thumb together, other fingers remain extended.

Benefits: heals, strengthens and balances the spiritual and physical body; regulates body weight; improves concentration, patience and complexion; reduces fatigue.

Shuni Mudra

a.k.a.: Shoonya/Shunya Mudra, Mudra of Emptiness

Position: tips of the middle finger and thumb together, other fingers remain extended.

Benefits: promotes alertness of the senses, relieves earaches.

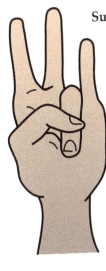

Surya Mudra

a.k.a.: Surya Ravi Mudra, Agni Mudra, Agni-Vardhak Mudra, Mudra of Fire, Mudra of the Sun/Earth. Some schools view it as being the same as Prithvi Mudra.

Position: fold your ring finger down so that the tip is touching the palm (or close to it), place your thumb over the ring finger, keeping the other fingers extended.

Benefits: improves eye health, vision, digestion, metabolism and cholesterol levels; increases body heat; reduces stress.

Vayu Mudra

a.k.a.: Mudra of Air

Position: curl your index, bringing the tip to the base of the thumb, press the base of your thumb back against your index, other fingers remain extended.

Benefits: helps to regulate ailments within the body resulting from an air imbalance: flatulence, bloating, arthritis; helps to reduce tremors in Parkinson's sufferers; reduces stress and anxiety; promotes clear skin.

Meditation

Have you ever felt the need to just chill out? Are you often being told that you need to relax? Do you find that you have a hard time wrapping your head around all the crazy things happening in your life? Do you feel that if one more thing gets added to your plate you're going to regurgitate unpleasantries on all those around you? Well, then, my friend, meditation is for you! All you need to do is find the time and space! Ha!

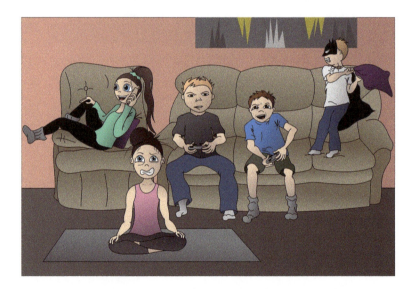

When taking on something new, most people need to know why they are doing it and what they are going to get out of it. Why am I going to the grocery store? To buy bananas. Why am I shovelling the snow from the driveway? To get my car out. Why eat enough fibre? To keep me regular. Why am I exercising my shoulders? To get cannonball delts. Why do we recycle? To save the planet. Why listen to The Backstreet Boys? Because they make me feel things. Why should I meditate?

Here's why.

Meditation:

Improves cognitive function
Promotes creativity
Boosts confidence and self-esteem
Improves memory
Provides mental clarity
Regulates blood pressure
Relieves arthritis pain
Reduces stress and anxiety
Boosts immunity
Improves respiratory system
Helps to recover from and fight addictions
Increases focus and concentration
Reduces inflammation
Promotes emotional stability
Reduces the frequency of mood swings
Increases energy levels
Improves problem-solving abilities
Gives peace of mind
Speeds up physical recovery caused by exercise, illness and injury
Decreases headache strength and frequency

Need I go on? I thought not.

Meditation 101: Quick Guide

Start small.
While a 30-45 minute meditation session might be your end game, you might want to start small. Meditation newbies may get bored trying to sit still for that long and struggle to get into and stay in that blissful state. Frustration can lead to giving up. Start with just five minutes a day. That's reasonable, isn't it? You've sat on the toilet for longer than that. Over time, as you get comfortable with 5 minutes, move up to 10 minutes. Keep increasing by 5-10 minute increments until you reach your goal time.

Find a time of day that works for you and stick to it.
You're busy, I'm busy, the whole world is busy. It's essential to take a step back from that chaos and schedule some "me time". Whether it's first thing in the morning, just before bed, over your lunch hour or on a coffee break, pick a time to start meditating. Since you're starting small, this shouldn't be too hard. To form a habit, it's important to set yourself a schedule to commit to your undertaking and hold yourself accountable. Set an alarm on your phone, make a date with a family member/roommate/co-worker, stick Post-its everywhere, whatever it takes so that when you're lying in bed at night, you're not wondering: wasn't there something I was supposed to do today? Once the habit is established and you're beginning to reap the benefits, you won't need the reminder. Meditation will be part of your everyday routine.

Set a goal.
It can be daunting to think that this is your life now. You must do this. Every day. Forever. There's no need to think that way until it's something that you *want* to do. Every day. Forever. Your perception of the task will change if you think of it as a challenge. Consider how many challenges you hear of, from going vegan for 30 days, to 7 days of minimalism. With an end in sight, there's no need to commit unless you really want to. Try to meditate every day for a week, or a month. Then re-evaluate and create a new

challenge if you want to. If you felt you weren't ready for meditation, stay committed to your asana and pranayama practice and then try again a little way down the road. No pressure.

Create your environment.
Find a quiet space with minimal distractions. Turn off your phone or leave it in another room. If there are people around, let them know what you're doing so that they don't disturb you. Dim the lights. Close the curtains. Set up a cozy spot in a clean area. Remember, the idea is to minimize distractions. If you're surrounded by a mess that you'll need to tidy later, your mind may drift to that. Get a zafu, zabuton, cushion or blanket to sit on. If you require a physical point of focus, light a candle or turn on a fake one for safety's sake. Wear comfortable clothing that doesn't irritate your skin or dig into your belly when you're seated. Do you need to pee? Let one rip? Get it done. How's your tummy? Inner environment is as important as outer. When did you last eat? A grumbling tummy is distracting. As is bloating from having eaten too much.

Choose a mudra.
Choose from the mudras listed previously, or have a go-to to keep things simple in the beginning. Sitting comfortably in an upright position, place your hands on your knees, palms facing up in your selected mudra, or folded in your lap in dhyana mudra.

Connect to your breath.
Begin by simply paying attention to how you're breathing. Slow it down and gain control of it. Breathe naturally with your belly protruding on the inhale and contracting on the exhale. Draw deep breaths through the nose, slow inhales, controlled exhales. Your exhales may be longer than your inhales, but not the other way around. Continue to focus on your breath until you begin to feel a sense of calmness.

Choose a point of focus.
Whether it's a physical point (the flame of a candle), a visualized symbol or place (a flower, a beach), a sound (ooooooooooommmmmm) or a mantra (using your inside voice or mumbled lightly), now's the time to concentrate on it. Focus.

If your mind strays, bring it back.
An itch on your nose, a car door slamming outside, the smell of coffee, your agenda for the day, something is likely to distract you. That's OK. As soon as you realize that you've strayed, return to your point of focus. If a negative thought has changed your breathing pattern causing it to quicken or become erratic, get that back under control before re-engaging your concentration.

Lose your point of focus.
As you become more relaxed and less susceptible to distraction, approaching the higher state of consciousness, allow your point of focus to vanish and simply concentrate on nothing. If you become aware, go back through your breath control (if required), then your point of focus until you return to a zoned-out trance.

Don't overthink it.
Don't be hard on yourself if it seems to be taking you a long time to get this thing right. Meditation seems simple, but sometimes it takes effort to make something effortless, the effort being your commitment to the practice, the control of your breath and concentration on your point of focus. You want to think about it until you don't have to think about it. Don't give up. One day you'll get it and you'll come out of it feeling like you're walking on clouds.

Keep a journal.
As I've said, we usually need a reason to do something. And we definitely need a reason to stick it out. Keeping a journal when you first start to meditate can help to encourage you to continue, or can help set a goal to improve what you've done in the past. It can be as detailed as you want, describing how you felt, before during

and after your practice. Or it can be as simple as using an emoji to portray the same thing.

Use the following pages as a guide to begin journaling a 7-day meditation experience. For a digital or downloadable version, visit:

>www.thecartoonyogi.com

MEDITATION *Journal*

ooooooooooooooooooooommmmmmmmmmmmmm

DATE:_____
DURATION:_____
MANTRA:_____

ooooooooooooooooooooommmmmmmmmmmmmm

MOOD BEFORE

_____
_____
_____
_____
_____
_____
_____
_____
_____
_____
_____
_____
_____
_____
_____
_____
_____
_____
_____

MOOD AFTER

MEDITATION *Journal*

ooooooooooooooooooommmmmmmmmmmmmm

DATE:_____
DURATION:_____
MANTRA:_____

ooooooooooooooooooommmmmmmmmmmmmm

MOOD BEFORE

MOOD AFTER

MEDITATION *Journal*

ooooooooooooooooooommmmmmmmmmmmmm
DATE:_____
DURATION:_____
MANTRA:_____
ooooooooooooooooooommmmmmmmmmmmmm

MOOD BEFORE

_____
_____
_____
_____
_____
_____
_____
_____
_____
_____
_____
_____
_____
_____
_____
_____
_____
_____

MOOD AFTER

MEDITATION *Journal*

ooooooooooooooooooommmmmmmmmmmmmm
DATE:_____
DURATION:_____
MANTRA:_____
ooooooooooooooooooommmmmmmmmmmmmm

MOOD BEFORE

_____
_____
_____
_____
_____
_____
_____
_____
_____
_____
_____
_____
_____
_____
_____
_____
_____
_____

MOOD AFTER

MEDITATION *Journal*

ooooooooooooooooooommmmmmmmmmmmm
DATE:_____
DURATION:_____
MANTRA:_____
ooooooooooooooooooommmmmmmmmmmmm

MOOD BEFORE

MOOD AFTER

MEDITATION *Journal*

ooooooooooooooooooommmmmmmmmmmmmm

DATE:_____
DURATION:_____
MANTRA:_____

ooooooooooooooooooommmmmmmmmmmmmm

MOOD BEFORE

_____
_____
_____
_____
_____
_____
_____
_____
_____
_____
_____
_____
_____
_____
_____
_____

MOOD AFTER

MEDITATION *Journal*

DATE:_____
DURATION:_____
MANTRA:_____

MOOD BEFORE

_____
_____
_____
_____
_____
_____
_____
_____
_____
_____
_____
_____
_____
_____
_____
_____
_____
_____
_____

MOOD AFTER

ELEVEN

Chaka-Chaka-Chakras!

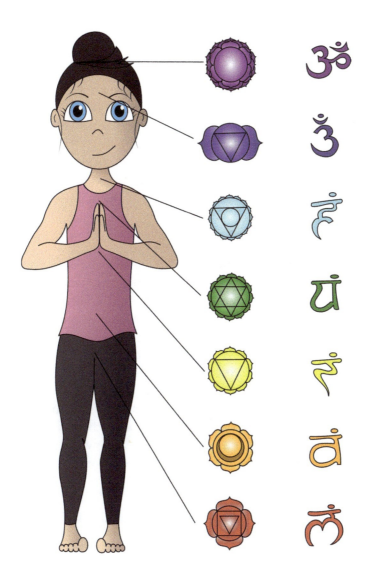

The chakras are subtle, swirling sources of energy within the body. Each is associated with a nerve centre located along the spine.

Through the practice of yoga, we can balance our chakras, keeping them open to allow energy to flow freely through the body. An imbalance or blockage of a chakra can lead to a dysfunction in the area of the physical body, and the emotional and spiritual characteristics, with which it is associated. Multiple techniques exist to open the chakras including asana, pranayama and meditation and going beyond yoga, through aromatherapy, colour therapy, crystals, etc.

There are seven chakras, beginning at the base of the spine and working up to the crown of the head. Each has their own set of characteristics, including a colour, a mantra sound, a planet, an element, a symbol, a lotus flower with a specific number of petals and more.

7- The Crown Chakra: (Sahasrara) The crown chakra is the source of consciousness that connects our spiritual and mental selves to the universe around us and to a higher energy. A balanced crown chakra is the ultimate goal of any yogi. Doing so will naturally align all of the other chakras, providing the practitioner with a sense of bliss. The crown chakra is blocked by egotism. It is naturally imbalanced because we are human. Imbalances: overactive = confusion, not living in the physical moment; underactive = a closed mind, spiritual skepticism. To balance: develop a spiritual practice, balance the other chakras, meditate with hands in dhyana mudra. / / / Location: crown of the head - Colour: violet or white - Mantra: (*silence*) Symbol: circle - Petals: 1000

6- The 3rd Eye Chakra: (Ajna) The 3rd eye chakra is the window to your higher consciousness. This chakra opens us up to possibilities and information that go beyond the physical world and our five senses. Being in tune with our 3rd eye grants us awareness and insight. It is countered by illusion. Imbalances: overactive = distracted by mysticism, does not live in the present, physical moment, delusions, obsessiveness; underactive = headache, lack of spirituality, insensitivity; To balance: engage in physical activity, walk barefoot, meditate with hands in dhyana mudra or prithvi mudra. / / / Location: forehead, between the eyes - Colour: indigo - Mantra: Aum - Symbol: a downward triangle within a circle - Petals: 2

5- The Throat Chakra: (Vishuddha) The throat chakra is that from which we emit our personal truths. It is from here that we may speak with wisdom and kindness. It is negatively affected by lies. Imbalances: overactive = speaking out of turn or inappropriately, often interrupting others, gossiping, mouth ailments; underactive = shyness, difficulty expressing oneself, digestive upset; To balance: think before you speak, meditate with hands in apana mudra or padma mudra / / / Location: throat - Colour: light blue - Mantra: Hum - Symbol: a circle within a downward triangle - Petals: 16

4- The Heart Chakra: (Anahata) The heart chakra is all about love and kindness for ourselves and others. It is connected to our health and ability to heal. It is impaired by grief. Imbalances: overactive = heart pain and regulations, codependency, jealousy; underactive = detachment from others, circulatory problems; To balance: practice self-love, treat yourself, meditate with hands in dhyana mudra or prithvi mudra / / / Location: Chest centre - Colour: green - Mantra: Yum - Symbol: a star made of two triangles - Petals: 12

3- The Solar Plexus Chakra: (Manipura) The solar plexus chakra is the hub of your willpower, self-confidence, conviction and inner strength. It is weakened by shame and is responsible for that intuitive gut feeling we get when something isn't right. Imbalances: overactive = anger, controlling behaviour, lack of empathy, digestive upset; underactive = insecurity, lack of energy; To balance: do something you know you're good at, meditate with hands in apana mudra or padma mudra / / / Location: upper abdomen - Colour: Yellow - Mantra: Ram - Symbol: downward triangle - Petals: 10

2- The Sacral Chakra: (Svadhisthana) The sacral chakra represents your creative identity. It is the force that drives you to find enjoyment in life. It is inhibited by guilt. Imbalances: overactive = addictive behaviour, hormone imbalances, obesity, oversensitivity; underactive = depression, decreased libido, fear of change; To balance: do some of your favourite things, meditate with hands in padma mudra or prana mudra / / / Location: just below navel - Colour: orange - Mantra: Vam - Symbol: upward crescent - Petals: 6

1- The Root Chakra: (Muladhara) The root chakra is your connection to the earth. It keeps you grounded and connected to the material world. It is associated with our overall sense of security, our survival instincts, career and financial independence. It is hindered by fear. Imbalances: overactive = anxiousness, overspending; underactive = daydreaming, lack of focus; To balance: spend time in nature, meditate with hands in prithvi mudra or surya mudra / / / Location: base of spine - Colour: Red - Mantra: Lam - Symbol: a downward triangle within a square - Petals: 4

TWELVE

Yoga Gear & Accessories

There was a time when all you needed to practise yoga, was you. Then props came into play, mats were introduced, the yoga pants craze barged into our lives and now, it seems we've got yoga accessories coming out the wazoo!

What do you need to start? (A mat and some clothes you can move around in.) What don't you need, but could find useful or fun? (So many things.) Some things you may already have on hand and others you may just want to skip altogether.

Apparel: From strappy tanks with built in bras to tight stretchy pants of all different lengths and colours, yoga apparel has become a multi-billion dollar industry. Do your pants actually need to be called yoga pants for you to practise in them? No. You can wear absolutely anything you feel comfortable in to practise yoga. Heck, you can wear nothing at all! (If you're at home alone or attending a Naked Yoga class, that is.) Be mindful of any dress codes at classes you attend and follow basic etiquette. Examples include: making sure your pants aren't see-through, and that their waistline sits above the line of your underwear or thong; if you're wearing shorts, make sure they won't show your crotch if you flip upside down; if your top falls over your head in inversions, make sure you have a proper bra on underneath (or tuck it in). Avoid long sleeves and thicker apparel if you're attending a hot yoga class. Try to wear clean, good-smelling clothes that are in good condition and provide minimal distraction to your practice and to the practice of those around you. There is no need to break the bank to feel and look good in a yoga class, where most people are focusing on themselves and not on you. Be warned, however, yoga clothes are addictive and as your practice grows, so will your ratio of athleisure wear to regular clothes.

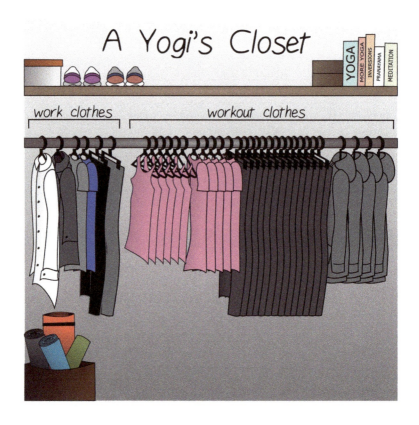

Blankets: While many types of blankets can be used to support your hips, knees, back and head during your asana, pranayama and meditation practices, there is a specific type of blanket that is used most often in yoga. A Mexican blanket, sometimes called a Yoga blanket, is made of a tightly woven fabric that is relatively thin as a single layer, can easily be rolled up and folds well to add height and cushioning as support. These blankets come in many different colours, and can be found everywhere online. They are inexpensive as far as blankets go, and if you

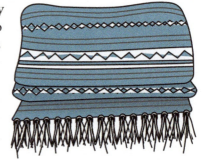

don't end up using it for yoga, it can be a pretty decoration for your living space.

Blocks: Blocks are a very popular and versatile prop in yoga asana, that can help you modify difficult poses to make them safer. They can also be used to challenge you, training your body for a more advanced variation. They aid in proper alignment and can help you find more height in arm balances. There are foam, bamboo, wood and cork blocks available, all at different price points and durability. Foam blocks are soft, very lightweight and will show indents and imperfections, which is fine for the price you pay. Be nice to mother earth and look for recycled foam. Bamboo and wooden blocks are made of natural materials and can be on the heavy side. They are very hard so if you plan to put some of your body weight into the block, they may be a bit uncomfortable. Cork blocks, also made of natural materials, are quite dense, making them a bit heavy, but they are not as hard as wood and bamboo, making them a bit more comfortable to use. Bamboo, wood and cork blocks all feel very stable, but are much pricier than foam blocks. Many yoga instructors will have blocks for the class to use, so there is no need to bring your own, unless otherwise specified. If you are developing a home practice, you can start without blocks, incorporating them if and when you want to. If you're not sure you would use them, you can try to use sturdy books in place at the beginning.

Bolsters: Yoga bolsters are long thick cushions used for support, modifications and to enhance relaxation. The shape of the cushion is what makes it more useful than just your average cushion or pillow for certain areas of the body, like along your spine, or behind your knees. A bolster could be interchangeable with a rolled-up blanket in some poses, and a regular square cushion in others. Like blocks, some studios have them on hand for you to use.

Chairs: Attending an Iyengar class, you're likely to see chairs in the studio for you to use. If you are practising at home and following an Iyengar video, a prop video or a chair yoga video, you'll want to have a chair ready before you start. Make sure that it is sturdy and that the feet won't slide. A regular kitchen chair or a folding chair will do. If you need padding on the seat of the chair, you can add a blanket or cushion.

Cushions: Cushions are great as props in yoga to elevate the hips for those with hip pain, lower back issues, and tight hamstrings. They can aid in relaxation and support you in meditation. Cushions are very useful to help the pregnant yogi practise safely and comfortably. Everybody is different and our preferences vary. You likely already have cushions (or pillows) at home, so start there and try a few out until you know what works for you. If you feel that using a cushion is essential to your asana practice, consider taking one to class with you, if there aren't any there for you to use. Just make sure before you do, however, that you know how and when to use it. A regular class is not the place to be asking your instructor for tips and instruction on using a prop that no one else is using. If that's what you need, look for a specialized class, take a one on one session with an instructor or find a video or book that can help you.

Essential Oils: Some teachers use essential oils in their class. Others may prefer not to due to sensitivities that some practitioners may have. Their many benefits may include: reducing headaches, stress and anxiety; increasing focus and mental clarity; improving respiratory and digestive function; and boosting the immune system. You can diffuse them at home to add to your practice, or apply them from roller bottles to pressure points on the body at home or before class. Just be sure that oils applied to the skin are diluted with a carrier oil first. Some brands are more expensive than others, mostly due to the quality of the oils themselves, but using essential oils does not need to be costly. By keeping just a few of your favourite oils on hand, you can create a variety of different blends.

The Cartoon Yogi's Go-To Oils

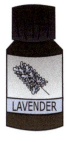 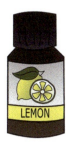 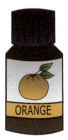 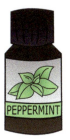 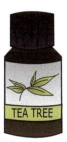

Grip Gloves: These are fingerless gloves with grips on the palms providing a non-slip surface to practise your asana anywhere you go. Great for travelling if you don't want to take a mat with you. These can be used as a temporary fix to provide extra grip on your mat, but to resolve this problem, you should be looking to get a better-for-you mat since the whole point of a yoga mat is to provide this support in the first place.

LED Candles: Flameless candles can be found everywhere now, providing the same atmosphere as wax candles without the fire. Scent-free environments are popular, and flameless candles are ideal for those. You can get some that flicker like a real flame and that turn on and off using a remote control. They help to create the ambiance you want, to encourage relaxation and meditation. Necessary? No. Pretty? Yes!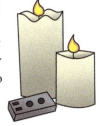

Mats: Since asana, as we know it, hasn't always been a part of the practice of yoga, the surface on which we practise has had to evolve over time to accommodate our sweet moves. Up until the 1980s, poses were either practised on a bare floor, or on a blanket or towel, which as you can imagine, did not provide much traction. Then, an English Iyengar yoga teacher named Angela Farmer stumbled upon a carpet underlay in the midst of her active search for something to solve this problem, that led to just that. Angela cut the material in the shape of a towel and began sharing it with other yogis. It was so popular that her father decided to retail them as "sticky mats". The underlay wasn't durable, however, so in 1990, a woman named Sara Chambers, founder of Hugger Mugger, created and manufactured a sturdier sticky mat, the first ever designed specifically for yoga. Since then, innumerable brands, styles, colours, patterns, thickness and materials of yoga mats have been created. The hard part now is finding the right one for you. Do you move with ease and like a quick practice? Opt for a thinner mat. Do you need extra support on hard surfaces? Look for a mat with a little more cushion. Is your home practice area carpeted? Go with a thick sturdy mat. Hot Yoga? There's a mat for that.

The prices of mats vary greatly. You can spend $5 at a dollar store, or over $100 on a designer brand. I wish I could tell you that you get what you pay for but yoga mat preference is a personal thing. I purchased a mat last year (mid-point price range) that multiple people swore by, and I *hated* it. I've used expensive mats that let you flow like an angel and some that were worthless. My favourite mat of all time cost about $20 in 2002 and has had a very good life. It's extremely worn now but I still use and love it. Ask around and read some reviews. If you're practising in a yoga studio, most will have mats that you can borrow and this may give you a feel for the type you want to buy.

Mat Bags: Mat bags are cylinder shaped sleeves with a strap on them that you use to carry your mat around. Some have pockets that you can put your keys and cards in which is useful if you're not carrying a purse or gym bag. Some gym bags have a section for your mat, doubling as a mat bag. And some gym bags are so big your mat fits right inside. So I guess those could be called mat bags too...

Mat Cleaner: Your body is going to be all over your mat. Including your face. Every now and then, it's a good idea to clean it. Your mat, not your face. Well, that too. If you have the label or tag that your mat came with when you purchased it, there may be specific cleaning instructions on it. Some mats can be placed in the washing machine. Alternatively, you may be able to wash your mat in the bathtub with some dish or laundry detergent. Whether machine washing or hand-washing, let your mat air dry draped over the tub, a shower curtain rod, or on a line outside. Make sure it is fully dry before rolling it back up, to prevent mould. For an everyday cleaner, you can buy or make a mat cleaning spray that you simply spritz onto your mat and let dry or wipe up after use.

DIY Yoga Mat Cleaner:
¾ cup water
¼ cup witch hazel or white vinegar
20-40 drops of essential oil

Combine in a spray bottle and shake to combine.

Essential Oil Combination Recommendations:
20 drops lavender + 10 drops tea tree
20 drops peppermint + 10 drops lemon
15 drops lavender + 15 drops lemon
15 drops peppermint + 15 drops orange

TIP: This spray along with one of the essential oil combinations above can be used before your practice to infuse your mat with a pleasant and calming (yet subtle) aroma that you'll love when your face gets down close to the floor.

Be warned, however, that smelling too close may transfer your makeup to your mat. I've done it. It's embarrassing.

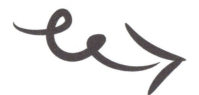 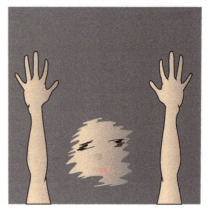

Mat Straps: This is a strap with loops or velcro at either end, used to slip onto your mat so that you can carry it around on your back. Some mats come with a strap when you purchase them. Some mat straps can double as yoga straps.

Music: When practising at home, it can get a little boring at first. Some people find music helpful and motivating. There are all types of music that are marketed to yogis, some for asana practice, and some for meditation, mostly instrumental, soft and calming. If that's not your thing, play anything that makes you happy. No one is saying you can't rock your practice out to ACDC.

Singing Bowls: Tibetan singing bowls have been used for thousands of years to aid in meditation and it is believed that the resonance they create helps to heal and balance the body. They are usually made with a combination of metal alloys, come with a striker and sometimes a cushion. To play a singing bowl, place the bowl on its cushion, or in the palm of your hand, being careful not to touch its sides. You can strike it like a gong or ring it around the rim. In a class setting, it may be played at the end of the class during savasana or relaxation. For home use, you can play it prior to meditation to still your body and mind, or even use it to calm down some crazy kids.

Straps: Yoga straps are a very popular and useful prop to add to your asana practice. Like blocks, they can help you safely modify a difficult pose, or deepen a challenging pose to help you advance in your practice. They are not just for beginners, they are for all yogis. Most will have a D-shaped ring at the end that you would use to create a loop. The loop should be easily adjustable so that you can modify it as you move through your practice to fit around your foot in one pose, then maybe your hips in the next. They come in multiple lengths, the longer ones being required for some techniques where the hips are involved. Since many yoga mats come with a mat strap that can double as a yoga strap, when gearing up, start with a mat already equipped with a mat strap, then look into yoga straps if you need to.

Towels: Towels are used in hot yoga (or a warm session where one might sweat a lot) to give you extra grip. They are usually the same size as your average yoga mat and made of a lightweight microfibre. You can use them to just wipe off extra sweat, or you can drape them over your yoga mat to stand on during the class. Unless you're planning on getting super sweaty, you don't need one. If you have unusually sweaty palms even in a regular class, you can bring a hand towel or a small microfibre towel (of the kind you might wash your car with) to place at the head of your mat for some slip resistance.

Yoga Balls: Yoga balls come in all different sizes with each having their own purpose. Some are small and designed for hand or foot rolling. Some are a little larger and help you to release fascia tension. Others, also known as exercise or stability balls can be used as equipment or props for core work. It is up to you whether you want to incorporate them into your practice. If they are being used in class, they will be provided to you there, unless otherwise specified. Specialized workshops might require a purchase of some sort. Some balls are marketed for use in therapeutic self-massage and are wonderful, but a tennis ball can do the same thing if you know where to roll it.

Yoga Socks: Compression socks, grippy socks, studio socks, there are a lot to choose from. You won't see a lot of people wearing them in class, however, as there is typically a specific reason why you would choose to wear socks during yoga asana. Meditation, sure! Go big and woolly. But for asana it's important to feel your feet on the mat. Those with circulation problems in their legs might wear compression socks. If you are always cold, there are socks that cover everything but your toes and heels. Grippy socks are just like grippy gloves, and can be used on any surface in place of a mat, so they are great for travelling.

You can also use them on your mat if grip is an issue.

Yoga Wheel: This is a relatively new prop that is used to release tension in the back, shoulders, neck, front torso and hips. It helps you to improve your practice bringing you more advanced and creative yoga postures in a safe and supported way. Like many other props/accessories, you won't need to buy one to attend class. Any class you attend that uses a yoga wheel will provide one for you (unless otherwise specified). Whether or not you use one at home is up to you. There are books and videos available to teach you how to use it.

YogaJellies: Another newish addition to the yoga world, this prop (that resemble breast pads) is a life saver for those suffering from carpal tunnel syndrome, arthritis, wrist pain, knee pain, flat feet or ankle issues. Supporting a portion of our body weight with our hands and wrists is very painful for some. And kneeling on a thin mat can be excruciating. Don't get me started on balancing on a flat foot. Extra stretching and rest between poses can suck up precious time when practising at home and is not always possible in class. While it is important to develop strength, resistance and techniques to help rid us of these types of pain, not every yogi has the time, patience or ability to do that. Jellies offer support and comfort to make your practice more enjoyable. *This is not an advertisement.*

Zabuton: A zabuton is a large square or rectangular cushion meant for sitting or kneeling. It originated in Japanese culture and was traditionally used by Zen Buddhists during meditation. Sometimes paired with a zafu, sometimes used to watch TV, zabutons are comfortable yet sturdy. If you have a hard time being comfortable in a seated position for long meditations and find the discomfort distracting, a large cushion like a zabuton might be right for you. Depending on the type of couch you have, you could use a sofa cushion instead.

Zafu: A zafu is a round cushion used in meditation to elevate the hips in a seated position. You would do this if you are tight or injured in the hips, knees or lower back, or if this is just a more comfortable position for you. It can be used alone, or rested on a zabuton.

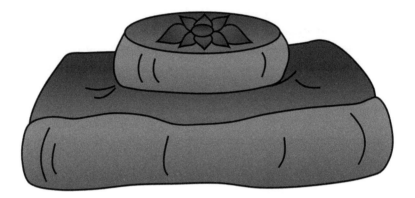

THIRTEEN

Five Weird Things Yogis Say

1. Breathe into your (insert body part here).
You will often hear a yoga teacher tell you to breathe into a specific part of your body. When it's your lower abdomen, or chest, then OK, we get it. But when you hear "breathe into your heels" or "breathe into your hips", what does it *meeeeaaaan*!? For example, while resting in Child's Pose, the breathing cue can be "breathe into your lower back". Your teacher wants you to bring awareness, and imagine the breath (or life force, or energy) flowing there to release tension in that area of the body.

2. Feel your body melt into the mat.
"Melting" the body into the mat, means to release all tension and allow gravity to pull your weight down without resistance so that you feel heavy on the mat. In Savasana, for example, your teacher may cue you to melt a specific part of the body or the whole body into the mat. What they mean is to focus on that part of the body, to notice if you are holding any tension there (flexing or lifting) and to relax it. When a teacher tells you to melt your heart into the mat, they are referring to the whole chest area, as well as any stress or emotions that may be weighing on you that need to be released.

3. Open your heart.
There is a physical and a spiritual side to this cue. Certain poses are great heart openers: Cobra, Camel, Bow, Sphinx, Wild Thing, etc. When you hear your teacher tell you to open your heart, they are telling you to widen through the chest. Or they may be using it interchangeably with "lift your heart" which means to lift the chest. Spiritually, this cue is a reminder to be compassionate, patient, kind and to welcome love into your life, releasing pain

and experiences that are holding you back emotionally. That's some deep stuff right there.

4. The four corners of your feet.
These refer to the ball under your big toe, the ball under your baby toe, and your inner and outer heels. Some yogis disagree with this structure and say that the foot does not have four corners, it has three corners forming a triangle: the balls under the big and baby toes and the heel. Either way, teachers use this cue to instruct you on where to put weight in your feet, whether it be to one side, or spread evenly across the whole foot. If you prefer one over the other, just picture it that way when you're practising. If you have very high arches, it may be easier for you to picture the triangle, so that your foot doesn't tilt inward. Yogis with lower arches can imagine the four corners to reverse their tendency to roll the feet inwardly by applying more pressure to the ball under the baby toe and the outer "corner" of the heel. It's your feet, you decide.

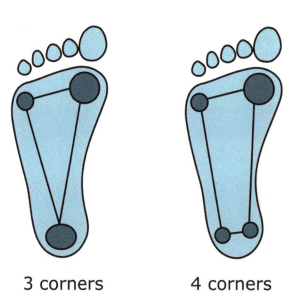

3 corners   4 corners

5. Float back/up.
From Standing Forward Bend, to Plank, to Downward Facing Dog, back to Standing Forward Bend...transitioning between these poses can be like a dance. As we gain more experience, strength and confidence as yogis, instead of stepping our feet back to Plank from Standing Forward Bend, or walking our feet up to Standing Forward Bend from Downward Facing Dog, we may want to jump back, or jump up. We see other yogis in the class doing it, especially when we're going through Sun Salutations. But the movement required here is not really a jump. Yoga is low-impact. Don't jump. If you jump back to Plank, or jump up to Standing Forward Bend, you can land hard and sometimes unevenly, which can send your joints out of alignment. And in yoga, we love proper alignment. Instead of jumping, you want to imagine you are floating and use as much core and upper body power as you can to land with as much control and as little impact as possible. Using the Float Back cue reminds us of that. Instead, your teacher may even say "give a little hop", which is their way of telling you to be cautious. Here is an example of the importance of this cue, of "floating" or "giving a little hop". Imagine you are hopping back from Standing Forward Bend to Plank. Your feet land hard and in that moment, you lose the engagement in your core, if it was even there to begin with, resulting in your belly dipping down and your lower back hyperextending quickly, without support. Do this enough times in one class and you may wake up the next morning barely able to get out of bed. The movement should have been slow and controlled, legs suspended momentarily as we guide them back to plank, our core remaining strong throughout. Note: while some practitioners believe that during a Sun Salutation, one should be floating back into Chaturanga Dandasana and not Plank Pose, it is cautious to go to Plank first, even for experienced yogis, as attempting to "land" in Chaturanga Dandasana increases the risk of injury since the alignment in the upper body for that pose is so specific.

BONUS WEIRD THING: That was a *juicy* hip opener!

Some yogis describe poses that feel particularly good as being juicy, yummy or delicious. (Insert eyeroll here.) I'm sorry, I can't jump on board with this one. I've never said it, I never will, writing it here was difficult but, to each their own. If you want to keep practising your yummy savasana, more power to you. Maybe we should start using food adjectives to describe poses that we don't like too. "My Forward Bend is mouldy, it needs work." "OMG, did you see her Chaturanga to Up Dog flow? It is so crunchy." "Girl, my Backbend is expired!"

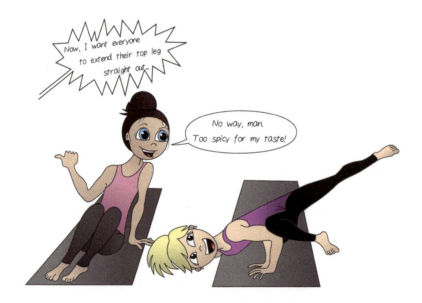

FOURTEEN

Eat Like a Yogi

Ayurveda

Ayurveda is an ancient form of medicine that uses food and lifestyle practices to keep its practitioners healthy. And since everybody is different, diet and lifestyle requirements will differ from person to person.

In Ayurveda, a dosha is the energy in the body that controls your physiology. You can find quizzes online to find out if you are predominantly one of three doshas: Vata, Pitta or Kapha. Each person possesses all three doshas within them, however, you will usually only have one that is the standout. This is the dosha that is present most of the time. Shifts in our routine and in our environment may bring forward our other dosha(s) while our dominant dosha retreats.

The Three Doshas

Vatas are typically thin and have difficulty putting on weight. They are nervous and anxious which takes up a lot of their energy. A solid routine is important to a Vata. They tend to be cold and have dry skin. When they are out of balance, they will be tired, anxious and constipated. In balance, they are alert and creative. Vatas have a delicate digestive system. They should consume warm foods that are easy to digest. Vatas should not participate in strenuous activity, and opt instead for low-impact, moderate forms of exercise like yoga, swimming, etc.

Pittas tend to be of average size and build and can easily maintain their weight. They are sharp, ambitious and focused. They possess an internal heat that makes them susceptible to anger. Because of this heat, they are often thirsty. When out of balance, Pittas will become frustrated, irritable and impatient. In balance, they are affectionate, expressive and intelligent. Pittas have a strong digestive system. They should consume foods that are cooling and be careful to stay hydrated.

Kaphas usually are on the bigger side and gain weight easily. They have good physical stamina. Kaphas are wary of new experiences so it is important for them to be adventurous. When out of balance, Kaphas are prone to insecurity, overeating and jealousy. In balance, they are orderly, efficient and loving. Kaphas have a slow digestive system. They should consume light foods and avoid excess oil and sugar. Kaphas should aim to be very active and incorporate exercise into their daily routine.

Anna Yoga

The yoga of food. Yoga philosophy teaches us that our food choices impact our health, energy and well-being. Food can be responsible for our energy levels, strength, emotional stability and good health, or it can be the source of our illness, hindered function and mental disarray. In yoga, foods are divided into three categories:

1- **Sattvic** foods include fresh fruits and vegetables, beans, legumes, almonds, dates, turmeric, ginger, cinnamon, natural sweeteners, whole grains, purified water, milk and butter. Sattvic foods are nourishing, giving us energy and mental clarity.

2- **Rajasic** foods include, eggs, some fish, processed sugars and flours, hot spices, chili peppers, onions, garlic, lemon, coffee, tea, spicy, and other sour, dry, bitter and acidic foods. Rajasic foods can be nutritious, depending on how they are prepared. Usually cooked up with oils, salt and spices, they are heavier and not as easily digested as sattvic foods. Rajasic foods can give us a boost of energy, making us feel temporarily strong and healthy.

However, they can create emotional imbalances and encourage depression, make a person restless and aggressive. Therefore, these are not foods we should be consuming every day.

3- **Tamasic** foods include meat, poultry, alcohol, fried foods, chips, foods preserved in vinegar or sugar, stale or underripe foods, processed foods, reheated foods and overcooked foods. Tamasic foods are difficult to digest. They slow us down, weaken us, make us lethargic and promote illness. They should be avoided.

Cleanses & Fasting

Cleanses and detoxes are practised in yoga to improve the digestive system and cleanse the body. They are often practised with certain poses that are helpful to "wring out" the organs and rid the body of toxins. Some go hand in hand with fasting, such as the Master Cleanse and other juice fasts.

Fasting helps to clear the mind and heal the body. It gives you an energy boost, mentally and physically. It purifies your soul. It helps to develop self-discipline. It has long been a part of the practice of yoga. Today, like so many other things, it's sort of faddish. There are many different kinds of fasts. If you choose to fast, it should be for the right reasons. Fast to mark a new beginning, or to find a better connection to yourself. Do it for the benefits it provides and not to deprive yourself of food for the sake of a diet. Yes, fasting can help you manage your weight, but it should not be your main reason to do it.

Eat Light

Practising yoga asana and meditation can be distracting and difficult if we feel full from our most recent binge. Eating light before your practice is a habit that is good to pick up. Yoga pants are tight enough as it is, am I right? If you're super hungry, wait until after your class to eat again rather than eating more before.

Believe me, you'll be more comfortable and content being able to forward fold without a bloated belly, or go into Child's Pose without clenching to hold in a fart. Avoid eating a big meal within two hours before a class, and anything at all within an hour before class, and you'll be good.

Hydrate

Dehydration negatively affects your energy levels, mood, sleep patterns, balance, strength and focus. It therefore goes without saying that proper hydration is essential to a healthy yoga practice. Aim to consume between 10 and 15 cups of non-caffeinated and non-alcoholic fluids per day. It doesn't have to be just water. Herbal teas, raw fruits and veggies and soups provide lots of hydration.

Compassion & Non-Violence

So we know that being a yogi does not mean that you have to be vegetarian or vegan. But also it does not mean that you shouldn't explore those types of cuisine from time to time. The choice is ultimately yours. As long as you feel good about what you are eating and it does not interfere with your physical abilities, proper digestion or personal ethics, then to each their own.

I once saw a meme of a girl saying, "I don't like vegan food, it's gross." Meanwhile, she was eating an apple. The joke, obviously, was that apples are vegan and yet she was enjoying one. The thing about vegan food as it relates to yoga is that as a yogi, you are encouraged to practise non-violence and compassion towards yourself and all other living things. This suggests that as humans, we should not harm animals by killing them for nourishment if we can find sustenance elsewhere. However, as a human, you are free to interpret the ethical standards of yoga as you see fit.

You are free to maintain your current diet, especially if you feel the way you eat upholds these standards. If you feel a disconnect between your yoga practice and your eating habits, that's OK too. Maybe you feel that as an individual in our society, you vote with your dollar and that every vote counts. So you choose to be vegan for health, or for ethical and/or environmental reasons.

You'll find that many yogis (and sometimes vegans) avoid the word vegan and prefer to call their way of eating plant-based. Why? Yogis practise self-care and like to be healthy...most of the time. Just because something is vegan, doesn't make it healthy. Oreos are vegan after all. Nothing against Oreos though...Oreos rock.

RECIPES

Here are some plant-based recipes that are sure to impress all your new yogi friends.

You'll notice that most of them yield large amounts of food. There are two reasons for this. The first is that yogis that yoga together, eat yoga food together. Your new friends may be a mix of vegan, vegetarian, pescatarian, omnivores and so on. Serving plant-based food that tastes great and will please everyone is essential when you get together to talk about yoga in your yoga pants.

The second reason is that as a yogi, you will now be devoting a lot of your time to yoga things, leaving you less time to worry about making food. Preparing these recipes in large quantities allows you to include them in your Sunday meal prep (something yogis love). This way, you have food for the whole week already made, leaving you more time to do yoga!

Tofu Scramble

A staple of vegan fare, it seems everyone has their own version of this delicious alternative to scrambled eggs. Tofu can be intimidating if you've never used it before. There are so many kinds! Just like yoga. Look for a non-silken, extra firm, organic, non-GMO variety. Sprouted is fine. Firm tofu is good too, if you can't find extra firm. Nutritional yeast, if you didn't know, is a fantastic ingredient with a nutty, cheesy flavour that can be used as a replacement for Parmesan and other cheeses. I think most people that are familiar with it though would agree that this ingredient should no longer be referred to as a substitute ingredient, since it's so good and nutritionally packed, it really does stand alone. Personalize this recipe by adding veggies of your liking such as mushrooms, spinach or peppers. Eat your tofu scramble on its own or in a western-style sandwich wrap. Yum!

Time: 30 minutes
Makes: 4 cups
Serves: 6

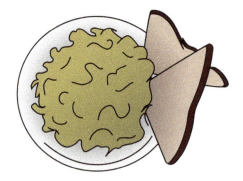

Ingredients:
1 tbsp oil
350 g extra firm tofu
1½ - 2 cups salsa
½ cup nutritional yeast
1 tsp yellow mustard
salt and pepper to taste

Directions:

1. Heat the oil in a pan over low-medium heat..
2. Crumble the tofu into the pan and add all remaining ingredients.
3. Cook for 15 minutes.

Sweet & Spicy Hummus

Honestly, I reduced the quantity of this recipe before including it here. In my house, we make four times this amount every week (we have a very large food processor). That much hummus will last our family of six about five days. Why? Because hummus is life. Eat this on its own with veggies and crackers. Spread it on toast or use it to replace the mayo in your sandwich. Mix some into your salad along with your favourite vinaigrette. Or combine it with salsa (half-and-half) for a vegan *queso* served with nacho chips. So good.

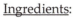

Time: 20 minutes
Makes: about 2 cups

Ingredients:
1 19 oz can chickpeas, drained, reserving liquid
¼ cup tahini
¼ cup lemon juice (or lime)
1 tbsp oil
1 chipotle pepper in adobo sauce (don't grab extra sauce, but don't shake any off either)
1 roasted red pepper (of the jarred variety, or roasted yourself)
2 cloves garlic
1 tsp sea salt (or to taste)
¼ tsp ground black pepper

Directions:

Add all ingredients to a food processor or blender and process, adding some of the reserved liquid from the can of chickpeas as needed (just a bit at a time) to get the desired consistency.

Note: If you run out of reserved liquid from the can of chickpeas or forgot to save some, you can use water instead.

Easy Tomato Soup

OK, I know canned soup is easier, but this soup really takes no time at all and it's so satisfying. For a fun variation, mix in a can of chickpeas with a couple of tablespoons of garam masala (to taste) and serve it over rice.

Time: 25 minutes
Makes: 10-11 cups

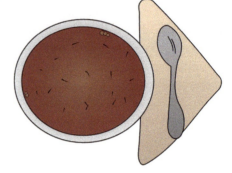

Ingredients:
1 medium onion, chopped
4 cloves garlic, crushed
2 cups vegetable broth
2 - 28 oz cans diced tomatoes
1 - 400 ml can coconut milk
½ cup nutritional yeast
1 tsp dried basil
1 tsp salt
ground black pepper to taste

Directions:

1. In a large pot over medium heat, cook the onion, garlic and ½ cup of the vegetable broth until the onions are clear, about 5-8 minutes.
2. Add remaining broth and all other ingredients, bring to a boil, then simmer for 10 minutes.
3. Blend with an immersion blender (or transfer to a food processor in batches) until smooth.

Rice Salad

Lunches for the week! This salad holds up well and is totally kid approved. It is great for parties and potlucks and sooooo tasty.

Time: 45-60 minutes
Makes: about 13-14 cups
Serves: 8

Ingredients:
3 cups rice, uncooked - about 9 c. cooked, white rice works best
1 large carrot, finely chopped, about 1 cup
½ English cucumber, peel on, finely chopped, about 1 cup
½ cup red onion, finely chopped
2 stalks celery, finely chopped, about ½ - ¾ cup
1 12 oz can corn, drained

Dressing:
1 large avocado
½ cup oil of your choice (I used avocado oil)
¼ cup water
¼ cup apple cider vinegar
¼ cup lemon juice
1 tbsp maple syrup (or sweetener of your choice)
1 tbsp Italiano-style seasoning
½ tsp salt
¼ tsp ground black pepper

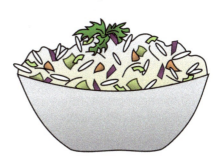

Directions:

1. Cook rice as per package directions and let cool slightly.
2. Use a blender to mix the dressing.
3. Combine the rice, vegetables, mashed avocado and dressing, and mix well.
4. Refrigerate & serve cold.

Red Lentil Curry Soup

This soup can be served on its own, or over rice for a filling meal. It is delicious and comforting with just the right blend of spices.

Time: 45 minutes
Makes: about 14 cups
Serves: 8

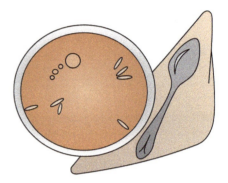

Ingredients:
¼ cup water
1 medium onion, chopped
4 cloves garlic, minced
1 tbsp fresh ginger, minced
2 tbsp curry powder
1 tbsp garam masala
1 tsp turmeric
1 tsp salt (or to taste)
¼ tsp ground black pepper
8 cups vegetable broth
1 400 ml can coconut milk
1 28 oz can diced tomatoes
2 cups dry red lentils

Directions:

1. Cook the onion in the ¼ cup of water in a large pot over medium heat until it starts to turn clear. Add the garlic and ginger and cook for two minutes more, stirring frequently.
2. Add all remaining ingredients and stir while bringing to a boil.
3. Reduce heat, cover and simmer for 30 minutes.
4. Serve alone or with rice.

Lentil Walnut Tacos

Oh yeah. Yogis love tacos. But who doesn't, right? This variety is simple and so good. Not to mention, it makes an awesome and impressive spread for a family dinner or a night with friends.

Time: 30-40 minutes
Makes: 12 tacos

Ingredients:
12 small corn tortillas or taco shells
1 tbsp oil
¼ cup onion, chopped
1 clove garlic, minced
1 19 oz can lentils, drained, not rinsed
1 cup walnuts, chopped
¼ cup vegetable broth
1½ tsp chili powder
½ tsp ground cumin
salt and pepper to taste

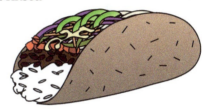

Suggested toppings:
salsa
shredded cabbage
thinly sliced red onions
chopped green onions
avocado
vegan cheese shreds
vegan sour cream
Tahini Lime Sauce (recipe to follow)

Directions:

1. In a large skillet over medium heat, cook the onions in the oil until they start to turn clear, add the garlic and cook for one minute more.

2. Add the lentils, walnuts, broth, chili powder, cumin, salt and pepper and cook for 10 minutes, stirring often.
3. Prepare the tortillas as per package directions (or wrap in foil and bake for 10 minutes at 350°F or 180°C - then separate right away so they don't stick together).
4. Add some of the lentil walnut mixture to the centre of each tortilla and add your toppings of choice.

Tahini Lime Sauce

This sauce is great on tacos, as a dressing for coleslaw, on a kale salad, with falafel, drizzled over a raw noodle salad, or as a dip for veggies. Remember, a little goes a long way. Adjust the ingredients and consistency to your taste and enjoy!

Time: 10 minutes
Makes: 1 - 1½ cups

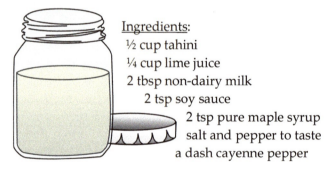

Ingredients:
½ cup tahini
¼ cup lime juice
2 tbsp non-dairy milk
2 tsp soy sauce
2 tsp pure maple syrup
salt and pepper to taste
a dash cayenne pepper

Directions:

Combine all ingredients. To make the sauce thinner, add a splash of non-dairy milk and stir. Repeat until you've reached the desired consistency.

Chickpea Cookie Dough

Who doesn't love cookie dough? And the classic combo of peanut butter and chocolate? Plus, a healthy dose of fibre to keep you regular? Sign me up!

Time: 15 minutes
Makes: 3 cups
Serves: 6

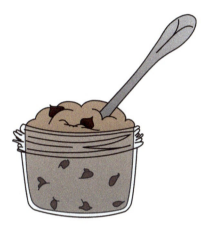

Ingredients:
½ cup quick oats, ground to a flour
1 19 oz can chickpeas, drained and rinsed
¾ cup peanut butter
3 dates, pitted
2 tbsp pure maple syrup
2 tsp vanilla extract
½ tsp sea salt
½ to ¾ cup mini semi-sweet or dark chocolate chips

Directions:

1. Process oats to a fine flour in a blender or the bowl of your food processor.
2. Combine all ingredients, except for chocolate chips, in the bowl of a food processor and process until smooth (about 5 minutes).
3. Dough may be warm from the processing. Allow to cool before stirring in the chocolate chips.
4. Chill, then serve as is, or with ice cream.

Banana Pudding

Wanna use up those overripe bananas? This dessert is light, sweet and creamy and an absolute perfect treat. Just try not to eat it all in one sitting!

Time: 15 minutes to prepare, plus 1+ hours to ready
Makes: 3½ cups
Serves: 7

Ingredients:
1 530 g package silken tofu, drained
2 ripe bananas, mashed
2 tbsp almond butter
2 tbsp pure maple syrup
1 tbsp coconut oil, melted
1 tsp vanilla extract
¼ tsp sea salt

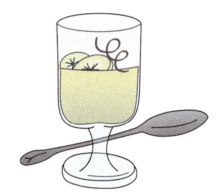

Suggested toppings:
banana slices
coconut whipped topping
shaved chocolate
sprinkled cocoa powder
sprinkled cinnamon
sprinkled nutmeg
chopped nuts

Directions:

1. Melt coconut oil.
2. Combine all ingredients in a blender and blend until smooth.
3. Refrigerate for at least 1 hour or until thickened.
4. Serve with toppings of choice.

Green Smoothie

This superfood, super tasty, super smoothie will make you feel like a superhero. Packed with goodness, this smoothie is nutrient rich and perfect for any time of the day.

Time: 15 minutes
Serves: 2 to 3

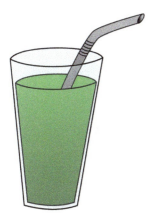

Ingredients:
2 bananas, frozen or fresh
1 cup frozen fruit blend of your choice
2 cups spinach, frozen or fresh
2 cups non-dairy milk
2 tsp spirulina powder
1 tsp wheatgrass powder
1 tbsp maca powder
1 tbsp flax oil
1 tbsp almond butter
Optional: 1 tsp pure maple syrup

Directions:

Combine all ingredients in a blender and blend until smooth.

FIFTEEN

A Yogi's Quick Guide

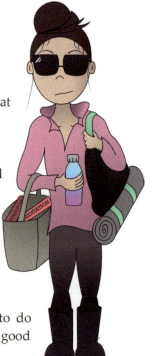

- As a yogi, you are never done learning.
- Practice compassion.
- Practice truth.
- Practice self-awareness.
- Practice self-discipline.
- Practice breathing techniques.
- Practice meditation.
- Try various styles, in class and at home.
- Practice safe asana.
- Know your body's limits.
- Comfy clothes and a mat are all you need to start.
- Poses aren't yummy, they don't taste like anything.
- Eat well.
- Eat light.
- Stay hydrated.
- Get a good night's sleep.
- There is always a reason not to do yoga, that doesn't mean it's a good one.
- Yoga makes your life better.
- Yoga is for everyone.

Acknowledgements

I would first like to thank my yoga teaching instructor, Tammy Abresch for her tips and guidance over the years.

I would like to thank my mother, Marguerite Lapalme Blais, for all the time she spent putting her excellent language skills to use in reviewing this work over and over. I promise, if there's a typo in this book, it's because of something I added after she played her part.

I would also like to thank some dear friends:

Julie Fox, my long time friend and fellow yoga teacher, for her input, tips, laughs, words of wisdom and time.

Brandon Lefebvre, for tolerating my incessant brainstorms, for reading through this book as a non-yogi, and for years of encouragement.

Katie Jorgensen, for her thorough proof-read and for thinking I'm funny, giving me the confidence to finalize this project.

Finally, I would like to thank my family. My husband & partner in crime, Denis, for his constant love and support, his assistance with my side projects (especially when I'm stuck and don't know how to proceed), his humour, and just for putting up with me in general. My children, Zoé, Jacob, Logan & Max for inspiring me, for their understanding when I want time to myself to draw cartoons and for doing so much adorable little yoga with me.

References

Books:

Adele, Deborah. 2009. The Yamas & Niyamas: Exploring Yoga's Ethical Practice. On~Word Bound Books, Minnesota. 192 pp.

Bachman, Nicolai. 2004. The Language of Yoga: Complete A to Z Guide to Asana Names, Sanskrit Terms and Chants. Sounds Truc Inc., Boulder, Colorado. 139 pp.

Barks, Coleman, translations by. 2004. The Essential Rumi. Harper One, New York. 388 pp.

Dias, Susie. 2004. Pranayama: The Path to Unlimited Energy. East to West Yoga, Toronto. 80 pp.

Dias, Susie. 2004. Raja Yoga: Taming the Mind for Inner Peace. East to West Yoga, Toronto. 88 pp.

Dias, Susie. 2004. Teaching Methodology I. East to West Yoga, Toronto. 68 pp.

Iyengar, B.K.S. 2014. B.K.S. Iyengar Yoga: The Path to Holistic Health. Dorling Kindersley Limited, revised edition, New York. 432 pp.

Karpel Oren, Goldie. 2013. Anatomy of Fitness: Yoga: The trainer's inside guide to your workout. Hinkler Books, Australia. 192 pp.

Judith, Anodea. 2003. Chakra Balancing: A Guide to Healing and Awakening Your Energy Body. Sounds True, Boulder, Colorado. 102 pp.

Lacerda, Daniel. 2015. 2100 Asanas. Black Dog & Leventhal Publishers, New York. 736 pp.

Prabhupada, A.C. Bhaktivedanta Swami. 2014. Bhagavad Gita: As It Is. The Bhaktivedanta Book Trust, Second Edition, Los Angeles. 873 pp.

Rost, Amy, compiled by. 2009. Natural Healing Wisdom & Know-How. Black Dog & Leventhal Publishers, New York. 496 pp.

Satchidananda, Sri Swami, translation and commentary by. 2016. The Yoga Sutras of Patanjali. Integral Yoga Publications, Fifth printing, Virginia. 252 pp.

Sears, JP. 2017. How To Be Ultra Spiritual: 12 ½ Steps To Spiritual Superiority. Sounds True, Boulder, Colorado. 251 pp.

Stephens, Mark. 2014. Yoga Adjustments: Philosophy, Principles, and Techniques. North Atlantic Books, Berkeley, California. 385 pp.

Stephens, Mark. 2012. Yoga Sequencing: Designing Transformative Yoga Classes. North Atlantic Books, Berkeley, California. 507 pp.

Surya Das, Lama. 1998. Awakening the Buddha Within. Broadway Books, New York. 414 pp.

Websites:

8 Limbs Yoga. About Yoga. [https://8limbsyoga.com/about-yoga/]. Accessed 9 February 2018.

Ananda Sangha Worldwide. Ananda Yoga. [https://www.ananda.org/spiritual-living/ananda-yoga/]. Accessed 13 February 2018.

Andreeva, Nadya. 2010. Ayurveda & Dosha Types for Beginners. [https://www.mindbodygreen.com/0-1117/Ayurveda-Dosha-Types-for-Beginners.html]. Accessed 21 March 2018.

Anusara School of Hatha Yoga. Methodology. [https://www.anusarayoga.com/methodology/]. Accessed 13 February 2018.

B.K.S. Iyengar Yoga. FAQs. [http://bksiyengar.com/modules/FAQ/faq.htm]. Accessed 12 February 2018.

Baptiste Institute. About Us. [https://www.baptisteyoga.com/pages/about-us]. Accessed 17 February 2018.

Bikram Yoga. About Us. [https://www.bikramyoga.com/about/bikram-yoga/]. Accessed 14 February 2018.

Bernstein, Susan. Yoga Benefits for Arthritis. [https://www.arthritis.org/living-with-arthritis/exercise/workouts/yoga/yoga-benefits.php]. Accessed 15 March 2018.

Brady, Adam. 10 Benefits of Restorative Yoga. [https://chopra.com/articles/10-benefits-of-restorative-yoga]. Accessed 16 February 2018.

Broga® Yoga. About Us. [https://brogayoga.com/aboutus/broga/]. Accessed 15 February 2018.

Carrico, Mara. 2007. The Branches of the Yoga Tree. [https://www.yogajournal.com/practice/the-branches-of-yoga]. Accessed 7 February 2018.

Carver, Leo. 10 Powerful Mudras and How to Use Them. [https://chopra.com/articles/10-powerful-mudras-and-how-to-use-them]. Accessed 26 February 2018.

Cosmic Kids Yoga. Kiersten. 2017. 8 Ways Kids Can Benefit From Yoga. [http://www.cosmickids.com/read/how-can-kids-yoga-benefit-my-child/]. Accessed 17 February 2018.

Dharma Yoga Wheel™. [https://www.dharmayogawheel.com/]. Accessed 6 March 2018.

Dangeli, Jevon. Tibetan Singing Bowls: The ancient brain entrainment methodology for healing and meditation. [http://jevondangeli.com/tibetan-singing-bowls-the-ancient-brain-entrainment-methodology-for-healing-and-meditation/]. Accessed 6 March 2018.

Do You Yoga. Sivananda Yoga. [https://www.doyouyoga.com/sivananda-yoga/]. Accessed 16 February 2018.

Do You Yoga. What is Kripalu Yoga? [https://www.doyouyoga.com/kripalu-yoga/]. Accessed 15 February 2018.

Eisler, Melissa. How and Why to Perform Bhastrika Breath. [https://chopra.com/articles/how-and-why-to-perform-bhastrika-breath]. Accessed 24 February 2018.

Ekhart, Esther. 2015. Cool down with Sitali Pranayama. [https://www.ekhartyoga.com/articles/cool-down-with-sitali-pranayama]. Accessed 24 February 2018.

Ekhart Yoga. Anusara Yoga. [https://www.ekhartyoga.com/more-yoga/yoga-styles/anusara-yoga]. Accessed 13 February 2018.

Ekhart Yoga. The benefits of Yin yoga. [https://www.ekhartyoga.com/articles/the-benefits-of-yin-yoga]. Accessed 17 February 2018.

Eliot, Travis. 2012. 8 Limbs of Yoga - A Brief Overview. [https://www.mindbodygreen.com/0-6391/8-Limbs-of-Yoga-A-Brief-Overview.html]. Accessed 7 February 2018.

Expanding Light. What is Ananda Yoga®? [https://www.expandinglight.org/anandayoga/what-is-ananda-yoga.php]. Accessed 13 February 2018.

Fierer, Lisa. 2017. Tantra Yoga: A Guide for Practitioners. [https://www.gaia.com/article/what-is-tantra-yoga]. Accessed 17 February 2018.

Fierer, Lisa. 2016. What is Kundalini Yoga? [https://www.gaia.com/article/what-is-kundalini-yoga]. Accessed 14 February 2018.

Fondin, Michelle. What Is a Chakra? [https://chopra.com/articles/what-is-a-chakra]. Accessed 1 March 2018.

Gabriel, Roger (Raghavanand). The 4 Paths of Yoga. [https://chopra.com/articles/the-4-paths-of-yoga]. Accessed 8 February 2018.

Godwin, Richard. 2017. 'He said he could do what he wanted': the scandal that rocked Bikram yoga. [https://www.theguardian.com/lifeandstyle/2017/feb/18/bikram-hot-yoga-scandal-choudhury-what-he-wanted]. Accessed 14 February 2018.

Graham, Caroline. 2016. Find me the yoga guru's Ferraris: British woman wins control of yogi Bikram's empire and 43 luxury cars after sex case...but they've vanished. [http://www.dailymail.co.uk/news/article-4078878/Find-yoga-guru-s-Ferraris-British-woman-wins-control-yogi-Bikram-s-empire-43-luxury-cars-sex-case-ve-vanished.html]. Accessed 14 February 2018.

Gupta, Soumya. 2016. Yoga: The Multibillion Dollar Industry. [http://bwdisrupt.businessworld.in/article/Yoga-The-Multibillion-Dollar-Industry/21-06-2016-99432/]. Accessed 5 March 2018.

Hugger Mugger™ Yoga Products. 2014. Yoga Mat History 101. [https://www.huggermugger.com/blog/2014/yoga-mat-history/]. Accessed 5 March 2018.

Imparato, Lauren. 2014. Bandhas for Beginners: Intro to Yoga's Interior Locks. [https://www.mindbodygreen.com/0-2583/Bandhas-for-Beginners-Intro-to-Yogas-Interior-Locks.html]. Accessed 25 February 2018.

Iyengar Yoga Canada. What is Iyengar Yoga. [https://www.iyengaryogacanada.com/iyac/what-iyengar-yoga]. Accessed 12 February 2018.

Jivamukti Yoga®. The Jivamukti Method. [https://jivamuktiyoga.com/the-jivamukti-method/]. Accessed 14 February 2018.

Kapanen, Kaisa. 7 Common Yoga Mudras Explained. [https://www.doyouyoga.com/7-common-yoga-mudras-explained-23667/]. Accessed 26 February 2018.

Keyes, Hilary. 2016. Japanese Encyclopedia: Zabuton (floor cushion). [https://matcha-jp.com/en/2503]. Accessed 6 March 2018.

Kundalini Yoga. Fundamentals of Kundalini Yoga. [http://www.kundaliniyoga.org/Fundamentals]. Accessed 14 February 2018.

Live and Dare. Giovanni. Scientific Benefits of Meditation - 76 Things You Might Be Missing Out On. [https://liveanddare.com/benefits-of-meditation/]. Accessed 29 February 2018.

McCall, Timothy. 2007. 38 Health Benefits of Yoga. [https://www.yogajournal.com/lifestyle/count-yoga-38-ways-yoga-keeps-fit]. Accessed 5 February 2018.

Macklin, Karen. 2014. AcroYoga Decoded: Grab a Yoga Partner and Go. [https://www.yogajournal.com/poses/acroyoga-decoded-grab-yoga-partner-go]. Accessed 12 February 2018.

Matthews, Kayla. 2015. Why You Should Try Aerial Yoga. [https://www.huffingtonpost.com/kayla-matthews/why-you-should-try-aerial-yoga_b_7258936.html]. Accessed 12 February 2018.

Mindvalley. 2017. The Complete Guide to the 7 Chakras: For Beginners. [https://blog.mindvalley.com/7-chakras/]. Accessed 1 March 2018.

Mordini, Silvia. Dirgha Pranayama and the Alchemy of Breath. [https://www.doyouyoga.com/dirgha-pranayama-and-the-alchemy-of-breath-79953/]. Accessed 23 February 2018.

Newlyn, Emma. 2016. 6 Branches of Yoga. [https://www.ekhartyoga.com/articles/the-6-branches-of-yoga]. Accessed 7 February 2018.

Pizer, Ann. 2018. Power Yoga Emphasizes Strength and Flexibility: Yoga Fit for the Gym. [https://www.verywellfit.com/what-is-power-yoga-3566853] Accessed 16 February 2018.

Saraswati, Dr. Swami Shankardev. 2011. [https://www.bigshakti.com/definitions-of-yoga/]. Accessed 7 February 2018.

Sivananda.org. 12 Basic Asanas. [https://www.sivananda.org/teachings/asana/12-basic-asanas.html]. Accessed 16 February 2018.

Stanger, Michelle. Common Mudras, Their Meaning, and How to Practice Them. [https://www.yogiapproved.com/om/common-mudras-meaning-practice/]. Accessed 27 February 2018.

Swenson, David and Gilgoff, Nancy. 2012. A brief history of yoga mats. [https://theconfluencecountdown.com/2012/03/29/a-brief-history-of-yoga-mats/]. Accessed 5 March 2018.

The Art of Living. The benefits of meditation you never knew. [https://www.artofliving.org/ca-en/benefits-meditation-you-never-knew]. Accessed 29 February 2018.

The Secrets of Yoga. What is Sivananda Yoga? Philosophy. Practice. [https://www.thesecretsofyoga.com/Sivananda/what-is-sivananda-yoga.html] Accessed 16 February 2018.

Thompson, Irene. 2016. Sanskrit. [http://aboutworldlanguages.com/sanskrit]. Accessed 16 February 2018.

Tweed, Katherine. 6 Yoga Poses That Age Well. [https://www.webmd.com/healthy-aging/features/yoga-for-seniors#1]. Accessed 17 February 2018.

Yoga Basics. Practice: Yoga Postures. [http://www.yogabasics.com/practice/yoga-postures/]. Accessed 25 February 2018.

Yoga Journal. Editors. 2007. Breath Retention. [https://www.yogajournal.com/poses/breath-retention]. Accessed 23 February 2018.

Yoga Journal. Poses. [https://www.yogajournal.com/poses]. Accessed 24 February 2018.

Yoga Journal. Editors. 2007. Style Profile: Kripalu Yoga. [https://www.yogajournal.com/yoga-101/spotlight-on-kripalu-yoga]. Accessed 15 February 2018.

Yoga Outlet. Guides: Poses & Sequences. [https://www.yogaoutlet.com/guides/poses-and-sequences]. Accessed 24 February 2018.

Yoga Outlet. How to Practice Kapalabhati Pranayama in Yoga. [https://www.yogaoutlet.com/guides/how-to-practice-kapalabhati-pranayama-in-yoga]. Accessed 23 February 2018.

Yoga Point. Pranayama - Breathing Exercises. [http://www.yogapoint.com/info/pranayama.htm]. Accessed 23 February 2018.

ABOUT THE AUTHOR

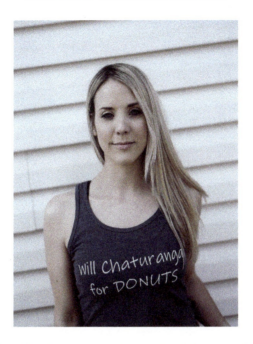

Krystel Dallas Houle is a yogi who works full time at her day job, has four kids, teaches yoga and other fitness classes part-time, attends yoga and other fitness classes as a student, runs a lot, sleeps occasionally, eats every chance she gets, creates videos for her YouTube channel (Krystel Dallas) and in her "spare" time, draws ridiculous cartoons.

She holds an EWYT-350hr & RYT-200hr yoga teaching designation, is a certified Yoga Exercise Specialist, a certified Pilates Mat Instructor, a Personal Training Specialist with additional studies in running coaching and foam rolling techniques.

She has been practicing yoga and Pilates since 2003 and has been teaching both since 2016.

CPSIA information can be obtained
at www.ICGtesting.com
Printed in the USA
BVHW021908010320
573750BV00014B/338